D1558083

Paleo Pasta!

The Art of Making Amazing Paleo, Grain-Free, and Gluten-Free Pasta

By

Dr. Danielle West- Stellick, ND

Unless otherwise disclosed, any advice relating to medical or nutritional advice, and Dr. Danielle West-Stellick, ND takes no responsibility for any consequences resulting from following such advice. You are solely responsible for any nutritional, medical, or dietary decisions you make.

ISBN: 978-1-887219-48-8

Published in the United States of America

Dedication

This book is dedicated to my wonderful husband, my loving Godly partner and best friend, who lovingly is reaping the culinary rewards of being married to an amateur chef and Paleo sleuth. I'd be lost without you!

Table of Contents

Introduction

One of my first naturopathic clients some 18 years ago was a sweet young Italian woman. As I was guiding her through dietary and nutritional changes and recommendations, when it came to suggesting she remove wheat from diet her, her immediate response was "But I'm Italian! How can you take pasta away from me?! What am I going to do?" Needless to say, she was quite distressed at the thought of a pasta-free future!

Similarly, at that time, there were no gluten-free pastas on the market. However, spelt, rice or corn, are the typical ingredients in some of the alternative gluten-free pasta which have since come to market. These of course are not acceptable foods on the Paleo diet; although they were the gluten-free pastas I was eating for many years once available. I even used to make a combination spelt and rice-based pasta from scratch.

Fast forward 15 years, and I was focusing on the Paleo diet and recommending it to others as well. Pasta seemed to suddenly be limited to spiralized vegetables; and I went through three types of spiralizing equipment: the small hand-held unit that looked like an hour glass with slicing blades on the side; a counter top unit with four sizes of slicing blades that required cranking the vegetable on a spindle, and finally I bought a higher priced spiralizer KitchenAid attachment. Spiralizing was fun, healthy, allowed me to be creative – but I wasn't thrilled at being pasta-less. Mac N Cheese with a non-dairy cheese and vegetables just doesn't provide the same satisfaction that real pasta does, even with a non-dairy Paleo cheese.

Enter PALEO PASTA, *real grain-free pasta*, and my life felt like I was given a new gift. Comfort food was back in my life!

But – truth be told, I quickly learned that unlike many other areas of cooking where you follow a recipe and you have a consistent result; making pasta had its own subtle nuances and required one to develop their own sense of the feel, taste, and texture and assure their ability to adjust the feel and texture of the raw dough on a batch by batch basis, as well as how to know if you have the right texture from the start just by looking at the ingredients. This was a skill I realized that I had now that I've been making one or two batches of Paleo Pasta weekly for over two years. I can look at the eggs, for example, as soon as they're cracked into a mixing bowl and know whether it would yield the perfect pasta dough or whether I would need to add additional starch or liquid to achieve the right texture literally from the start.

I've also made pasta by completely hand, by machine, and by hand preparation subsequently rolling and slicing with the KitchenAid pasta attachments. Each carry with it a different ease of ability to modify the ingredients as required during the preparation phase. Thus, I feel I'm in a position to discuss the pros and cons of various pasta machines as well as appliances, attachments, and tools.

Finally, I took my pasta recipe and looked at all the pasta-bilities – which were endless and have savory and sweet meal sections and desserts, plain and flavored pastas, and sauces galore!

I welcome you to join me on an exciting journey as I introduce you to the endless pasta-bilities of Paleo Pasta!

Chapter One: Sharing an Experience

Here's just a little pasta motivation. Mind you, I've been making Paleo pasta from scratch for about 2 ½ years. But as you go through the recipes in this book, especially the first few chapters on making the actual pasta and you have your successes and failures, it is my hope that this story should serve as a reminder of why, once you keep at it, this book and making your own Paleo Pasta will become something that you can't get anywhere else!

In addition to maintaining a Paleo diet when out of the house and at restaurants, because of medical reasons, I have to be rigidly gluten-free. Luckily, my husband's company Christmas Party this year was held at one of the few restaurants in town that understand the importance of food prep and handling when serving gluten-free items; have a solid menu with over half gluten-free; separate prep area, etc. So, I felt comfortable eating there, reminding the server of my gluten-free needs relative to food preparation and food handling, especially since our group was rather large and dishes/plates and other items could easily get mixed up.

One of the items that was prepared in their separate gluten-free area was Sinatra Chicken. Unbeknownst to me, it came with the chicken on a bed of GF pasta. In typical fashion, I still pushed the pasta aside and focused my energy on the chicken. Well, curiosity got the better of me and I very tentatively tried a bit of the pasta. RICE AND WATER! UGH!!! BLECH!!! My husband just cracked up!!!

But that's actually the state of so much of the gluten-free pastas – the majority tastes like cardboard or worse, especially if it doesn't have corn meal or another gluten-free bean flour in it. I can't tell you how many gluten-free pastas we tried over the years before going Paleo.

Of course, typically, people think of pasta as the filler to go with a sauce so it doesn't have to have much flavor of its own -- how wrong! Pasta can be, and should be delicious and stand on its own!

Then of course, we went Paleo. Initially, we thought all traditional pastas were a thing of the past, and I invested heavily in a series of spiralizers. Vegetables, which of course are very healthy, became our pasta for many months. But this kitchen sleuth, and admitted pasta-holic, still felt something was missing.

Enter Paleo Pasta. On someone's blog, I heard about a company that made Paleo Pasta and offered direct shipping. I was over the moon! I looked at their website, discussed the expense with my husband, and we ordered with great expectations. Out of four packages, only one arrived without damage; the hard plastic shells on all other packaging was crushed, with pieces and shards of the plastic embedded in the dried-out pasta that had molded. I was devastated. Although they sent replacements, they arrived in the same damaged condition. I was not happy, to say the least. But – the Paleo Pasta from one package that I was able to salvage from the original order was very hearty and I enjoyed it. Not exactly light or delicate as pasta should be, but it was Paleo Pasta and I enjoyed the flavor profile (key part of the story) so I was still happy!

When I go grocery shopping, especially at health oriented grocery stores, I wander the isles to see if any new Paleo items have come in. Low and behold I saw the same company's line of Paleo Pasta offerings in a refrigerated section. But what did my keen consumer's eyes find just going through the packages? The majority were molded!!! When I found a package on the shelves that was not moldy, it molded within a day at home. I was not amused, especially at those prices.

I decided it was time for me to put my Paleo kitchen sleuth hat on and investigate. It couldn't be that hard to make, right? After all, I already used and always stocked the basic ingredients.

And thus, the journey began... and continued and evolved and we enjoy Paleo Pasta dishes ranging from appetizers to meals to desserts fresh made several times a week! As will be highlighted through the recipes for pastas as well as dishes, ingredients ranged from basic to the more exotic including sweet potato flour, tomato powder, spinach powder, and beet powder to coffee flour, cocoa powder, banana flour, and strawberry flour. My journey has evolved from hand mixing and hand rolling pasta to using various automated pasta makers to using pasta rollers and cutters and other tools.

What I did learn and what has been continually reinforced over the last several years of making my own Paleo Pasta is how easy it really is to make! And of course, it's ALL inherently gluten- and grain-free!

And so, this book was born. There is no reason not to enjoy real pasta just because you're on a Paleo diet. And, as I'm very fond of saying to people when they believe anything gluten-free, especially grain-free or Paleo, just tastes like cardboard or worse, "You haven't tasted my cooking!" And now, it can be your cooking too! To me, this is just another reminder of how badly this book is needed!

Following on the footsteps of the rave reviews I'm getting on the recipes in my Paleo Basics book, this book is your opportunity to become a Paleo, grain-free, and gluten-free pasta PRO!

Chapter Two: Texture

Although I adore each and every recipe in this book, to me, this chapter is the key to making amazing Paleo, grain-free, and gluten-free pasta – you see, it's all about texture!

When you read a typical recipe and it calls for two or three large eggs, it's almost as if the recipe creator assumes that all eggs graded a specific size are created equal across all chickendom. However, the reality is that all large eggs, for example, do not contain the exact same size yolk or amount of egg white. In defense of the recipe creator, typically it really won't matter if there is 1/8 of a teaspoon more yolk or egg white in one egg when compared to another used in the same recipe. This rule, however, is NOT the case when it comes to making Paleo, grain-free, and gluten-free pasta! I cannot emphasize this enough.

To be honest, when I started making gluten-free pasta before I began following a Paleo diet, it was the same way – I was completely ignorant of how important dough texture was in regards to the specific amounts of each ingredient called for. I had mushy gluten-free pasta and I had very dense, tough, and heavy gluten-free pasta. It was the same when I switched to a Paleo diet and cooking. For each recipe, I was simply following a recipe or the creating one based on conversions to grain-free, gluten-free or Paleo ingredients. After all, how hard could it really be, I thought. You see chefs on television whipping off pasta in no time at all and with the greatest of ease... Texture my friend, texture.

And that is not typically discussed in recipes.

So, I pondered how I was going to tangibly relate what that perfect texture is that you are looking to achieve when making your own Paleo pasta, and then I found it.

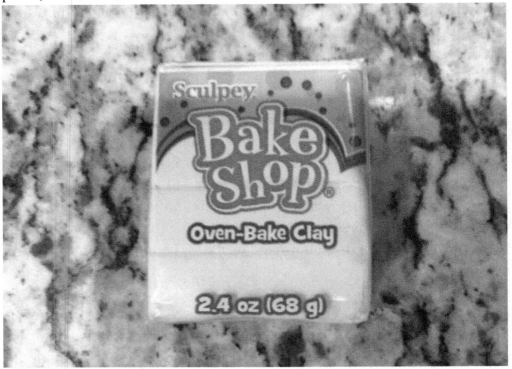

The perfect Paleo, grain-free, and gluten-free pasta dough texture that you are trying to achieve can be felt tangibly!

There is this handy dandy little product you can find in craft stores or even Walmart in the craft section for less than a dollar: Sculpey Bake Shop Oven-Bake Clay. Note: I do not believe all oven-bake clays are the same, so I cannot vouch for any other product that Sculpey Bake Shop's clay.

Now, when you open you package, the feel of the clay will seem awfully hard and dense. That is NOT the texture you are looking for.

But this is: Open your oven-bake clay, and pinch off a tiny piece about the size of the tip of your finger. Then knead it by folding it over on itself three times – you'll feel it soften and become more pliable, but you'll notice it is not too soft or gummy feeling. This is the texture you are trying to emulate in your perfect Paleo, grain-free, or gluten-free pasta!

I hope this brief chapter helps!

Chapter Three: Equipment

My experiences in coming up with just the right combination of pasta-making equipment that *works for me* has been an evolutionary process. In order to help you along your Paleo, grain-free, and gluten-free pasta making journey, I thought I'd share some of my experiences.

Making the pasta dough itself can be divided into three categories:
1. Completely manual
2. Mixed manual and tools
3. Completely automatic

I'll discuss each of these separately.

However, for each of these, you'll still need a large pot with rapidly boiling spring or filtered water to toss your cut pasta dough into to cook. Anything cooler than rapidly boiling water can lead to pasta strands sticking together.

Completely Manual

To make pasta "the old-fashioned way" like grandma used to make (process wise), you will need the following:
- medium mixing bowl
- fork
- measuring cups
- parchment paper
- rolling pin
- sharp knife
- nitrile gloves (optional)
- and strong hands!

Options to the use of a knife include a standard pastry cutter with a single blade:

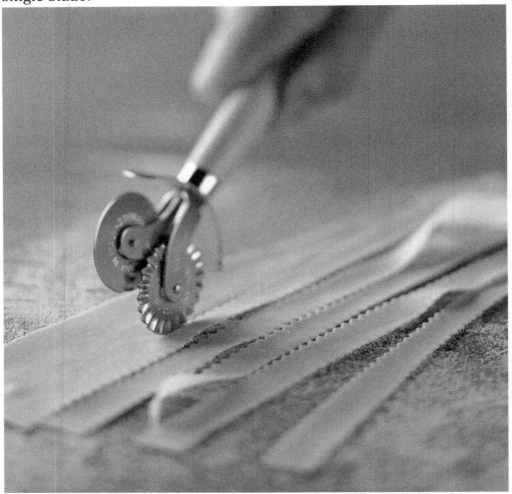

Personally, I like the Ateco multi-wheel pastry cutter by August Thomsen (available from Webstaurantstore.com) pictured next. This ensures that you have nice even and perfectly spaced pasta, and as the picture shows, you can adjust the width of the pasta strands to as wide or narrow as you prefer.

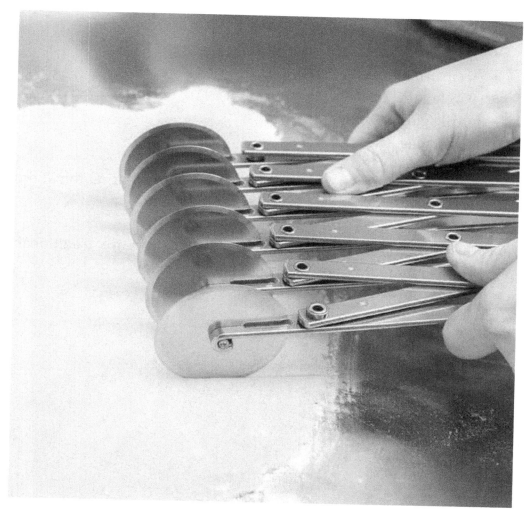

Mixed Manual and Tools

This is the method I'm currently using, as it allows me the flexibility of adding various Paleo flours or spices into the dough while assuring I achieve the proper texture. Then for rolling and slicing, I use my more tools. I stress, this is what works for me. I encourage you to experiment and find what works best for you!

You'll still need the same equipment for making the pasta dough itself:

- medium mixing bowl
- fork
- measuring cups
- parchment paper
- nitrile gloves (optional)
- and strong hands!

However, for the rolling and cutting, that's where the automation comes in!

There are a variety of options, for example, the more traditional counter top mounted version of a roller pictured below.

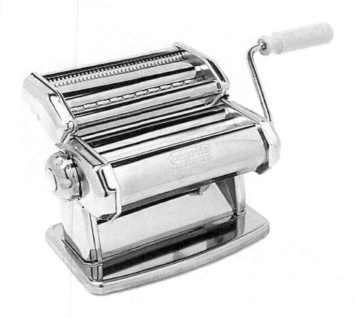

Pasta rollers and slicers such as this come in a variety of price ranges and are readily available from most home goods stores or departments. This is actually what I used many years ago when I began my pasta making journey. However, like using a rolling in, you do need a certain amount of strength to crank the machine.

Another option that is more automated, and personally is one I opted for, is the roller and slicer attachment that fits into my KitchenAid mixer.

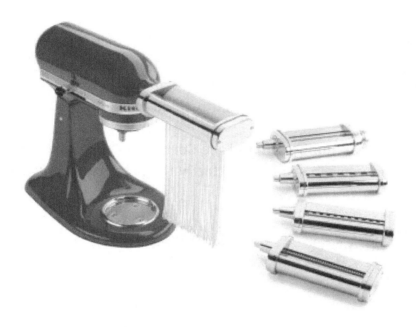

All I do is feed the dough in to the roller (pictured on the very top of the four attachments pictured on the left), using that process to further knead the dough by feeding it into the roller three times, and then feed it into a slicer. I let my KitchenAid do all the hard hand-cranking work.

Completely Automatic

Here's where the story gets interesting. We were in a well-known home goods store the year the Philips Pasta Making Machine came out, and it was on sale for $199. That plus a 20% off coupon for the store made it slightly more affordable for many, but still beyond our means at the time. Well, then I started making Paleo pasta on a very regular basis, strictly manual, and I'll be the first to admit, I'm not the best at rolling or slicing dough very evenly.

To that end, my sweet husband thought I definitely needed a fully automated pasta making machine. By this time the Philips unit had gone up to its full retail of $299; definitely not an option, 20% off or not! Thus, the quest for the perfect fully automated machine began!

For Christmas that year, hubby ordered the Gormia unit pictured here to surprise me. And you can see how perfectly the pasta came out the first time I used it!

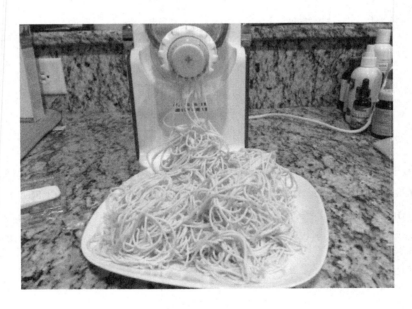

Most fully automated pasta makers function along the same basic principle: your ingredients go into the mixing bin, a blade or mixing roller mixes all ingredients together, and then the dough is caught up into an extruding roller which pushes the dough through a short chamber where there is a dough shape press at the end. In this case the press used was for spaghetti noodles. Most fully automated units come with up to 10 die casts for different pasta noodle options which range from spaghetti and angel hair pasta to linguini, lasagna, macaroni and more.

Now, I loved my Gormia unit. I was over the moon with it. However, the trouble with the Gormia unit was the chamber was small and I could only make half of my normal Paleo pasta recipe at a time, and I go through a lot of pasta!

Additionally, like other fully automated units, you can't feel the texture of the dough before it comes out of the extruder unless you stop the machine entirely first. Truth be told, the times I've done that and the texture is too soft or hard and I've added a few drops of water or a bit more of a Paleo flour-based ingredient in the unit itself, it's not mixed well unless I physically removed the dough, them mixed and kneaded the dough by hand and put it back in the automated unit before extruding. Of course, this pretty much defeats the whole purpose of having a fully automated pasta maker.

However, for those interested in a reliable and affordable fully automated pasta maker, the Gormia is the only one that means the unique mixing needs of working with grain-free flours! You absolutely have to knead the dough for five minutes, especially when working with almond flour due to the fats involved, otherwise the dough will not achieve the proper texture. The Gormia is the only fully automated unit on the market that will mix and knead dough for five minutes; all others only mix the dough for three minutes before automatically extruding the dough.

As my Paleo pasta making journey progressed and I was making several batches of pasta at a time, my husband of course, thought it was time we reinvestigate a unit with a larger mixing bin so that I could make one normal or larger sized batch at a time and be done with it.

We purchased several, including a Philips knock off made by with the same design specifications as the Philips. It leaked, didn't knead the dough for five minutes, and was a disaster! Others we tried had the same problem, they leaked! Upon reading reviews of these varied machines, low and behold, those who were dissatisfied with the units stated exactly the same thing – it leaked! The Philips knock-off also said it worked with gluten-free flours. Well, there is a difference between gluten-free and grain-free flours. Please, if you decide to look into purchasing a fully automated pasta machine, be aware of this one concept above all else: the machine must work to the specifications you need or it's not worth the money you will spend.

This is another reason that unless I use my Gormia, I typically use a combined manual and automated approach to making the Paleo, grain-free, and gluten-free pasta recipes in this book! I know exactly what I'm trying to achieve and most of the other fully automated pasta machines simply don't achieve the results for my needs!

Chapter Four: Basic Paleo, Grain-Free, and Gluten-Free Pasta

The basic Paleo, grain-free, and gluten-free Pasta recipe is very simple with five readily available ingredients: almond flour, tapioca flour, arrowroot flour, salt, and large eggs. That's it!

Now, before we get into the actual amounts let me make a few comments. You might be thinking to yourself, "Hmmm, tapioca flour and arrowroot flour can usually be substituted for each other in recipes, so why do I have to use both?" The short answer is simply because of the specific properties that each flour possesses.

The basic recipe is also one that, as you will see in the next chapter, mastering the basic recipe first opens up a whole world of pasta-bilities!

Basic Paleo Pasta Recipe
Ingredients:
½ C Ultra-fine ground almond flour
½ C Tapioca flour
1/3 C Arrowroot flour + ¼ C for final kneading
2 t Himalayan salt
2 Large egg yolks
1 Large egg

Instructions:
1. Prepare a large pot with boiling water. I usually pre-boil the water before putting it in the pot and then set the burner to achieve a rapid boil when I am at step 8
2. Prepare your workspace with parchment
3. Put on nitrile gloves

4. In a medium mixing bowl, blend together all dry ingredients (minus the ¼ C arrowroot used in the final kneading)
5. In a small ramekin, beat together egg yolks and full egg
6. Make a well in the center of the dry ingredients and pour egg the egg mixture in the center of the well
7. Using a fork, gradually blend in flour mixture into beaten eggs. (Picture drawing in the flour from the edges and working it into the eggs on a gradual yet continual basis)
8. When you cannot use your fork anymore, begin hand mixing and kneading of the pasta dough for five minutes
9. At the end of five minutes scatter the ¼ C arrowroot on your parchment and place dough on top of loose arrowroot. Knead additional arrowroot into the dough to achieve the texture discussed in Chapter Two.

At this point either roll to 1/8 inch on your already floured parchment paper by using a top sheet of parchment between your rolling pin and dough and slicing by hand or a pastry cutter, using a hand-crank roller and slicer, or use an automated roller and slicer. Once you have your sliced pasta, immediately toss it into rapidly boiling water for 5 minutes or until done to your particular texture tastes.

The picture in the last chapter (and on the cover) shows the basic Paleo pasta recipe cut using a spaghetti disk and being extruded from the Gormia before going into boiling water. The picture below shows the basic Paleo pasta recipe in a linguini cut (one of my favorite for some reason) freshly cooked! Contrasting the two, you can see the cooked Paleo pasta is much lighter in color. You'll notice this to an even greater degree when you start making the flavored Paleo pastas in the next chapter.

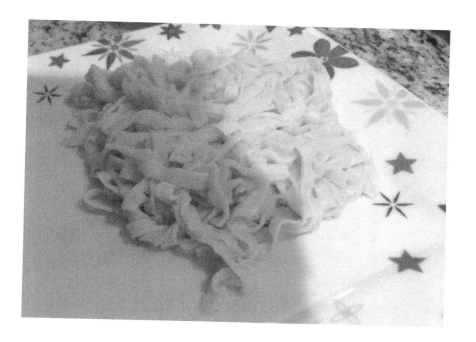

What About the Instant Pot?

Many readers use an Instant Pot and are avid fans of cooking with this wonderful appliance. I am no exception, I love my Instant Pot. HOWEVER, Paleo pasta is NOT Instant Pot compatible on recipes calling for including pasta in the pressure cycle, particularly if there is a sauce, such as beef stroganoff. The starches in the Paleo pasta will thicken your sauce in the instant Pot and it will not come to pressure no matter how much you try to thin the sauce with broth, stock, or other liquid you may have cooking with your other ingredients.

I strongly suggest you make your Paleo pasta as per the instructions here, boiling separately, then add already cooked pasta to your dish and gently stir. Or, use your Instant Pot to create your base meal, and serve the meal on top of plated Paleo pasta rather than mixing it together in casserole form.

Chapter Five: Sweet and Savory Pastas

Sweet Potato Pasta

Ingredients:

- 1 C Sweet potato flour
- 1/3 C Ultra-fine ground almond flour
- ¼ C Arrowroot flour for final kneading
- 2 t Himalayan salt
- 2 Large egg yolks
- 1 Large egg

Instructions:

1. Prepare a large pot with boiling water. I usually pre-boil the water before putting it in the pot and then set the burner to achieve a rapid boil when I am at step 8
2. Prepare your workspace with parchment
3. Put on nitrile gloves
4. In a medium mixing bowl, blend together all dry ingredients (minus the ¼ C arrowroot used in the final kneading)
5. In a small ramekin, beat together egg yolks and full egg
6. Make a well in the center of the dry ingredients and pour egg the egg mixture in the center of the well
7. Using a fork, gradually blend in flour mixture into beaten eggs. (Picture drawing in the flour from the edges and working it into the eggs on a gradual yet continual basis)
8. When you cannot use your fork anymore, begin hand mixing and kneading of the pasta dough for five minutes
9. At the end of five minutes scatter the ¼ C arrowroot on your parchment and place dough on top of loose arrowroot. Knead additional arrowroot into the dough to achieve the texture discussed in Chapter Two.

At this point either roll to 1/8 inch on your already floured parchment paper by using a top sheet of parchment between your rolling pin and dough and slicing by hand or a pastry cutter, using a hand-crank roller and slicer, or use an automated roller and slicer. Once you have your sliced pasta, immediately toss it into rapidly boiling water for 5 minutes or until done to your particular texture tastes. Unlike conventional pasta you'd find in the grocery store, and even some gluten-free pastas, I've not found the basic recipe go to "mush" from overcooking.

Spinach Pasta

Ingredients:

- ½ C Ultra-fine ground almond flour
- 1/3 C Tapioca flour
- 1/3 C Arrowroot flour + ¼ C for final kneading
- 2 ½ T Spinach powder
- 2 t Himalayan salt
- 2 Large egg yolks
- 1 Large egg

Instructions:

1. Prepare a large pot with boiling water. I usually pre-boil the water before putting it in the pot and then set the burner to achieve a rapid boil when I am at step 8
2. Prepare your workspace with parchment
3. Put on nitrile gloves (important when using fruit or vegetable powders as they will stain!)
4. In a medium mixing bowl, blend together all dry ingredients (minus the ¼ C arrowroot used in the final kneading)
5. In a small ramekin, beat together egg yolks and full egg
6. Make a well in the center of the dry ingredients and pour egg the egg mixture in the center of the well
7. Using a fork, gradually blend in flour mixture into beaten eggs. (Picture drawing in the flour from the edges and working it into the eggs on a gradual yet continual basis)
8. When you cannot use your fork anymore, begin hand mixing and kneading of the pasta dough for five minutes
9. At the end of five minutes scatter the ¼ C arrowroot on your parchment and place dough on top of loose arrowroot. Knead additional arrowroot into the dough to achieve the texture discussed in Chapter Two.

At this point either roll to 1/8 inch on your already floured parchment paper by using a top sheet of parchment between your rolling pin and dough and slicing by hand or a pastry cutter, using a hand-crank roller and slicer, or use an automated roller and slicer. Once you have your sliced pasta, immediately toss it into rapidly boiling water for 5 minutes or until done to your particular texture tastes. Unlike conventional pasta you'd find in the grocery store, and even some gluten-free pastas, I've not found the basic recipe go to "mush" from overcooking.

Tomato Pasta

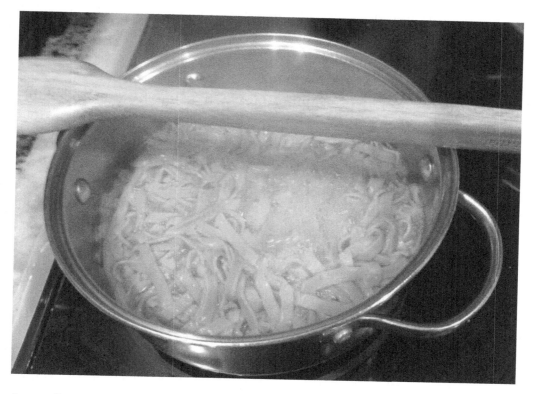

Ingredients:

- ½ C Ultra-fine ground almond flour
- 1/3 C Tapioca flour
- 1/3 C Arrowroot flour + ¼ C for final kneading
- 2 ½ T Tomato powder
- 2 t Himalayan salt
- 2 Large egg yolks
- 1 Large egg

Instructions:

1. Prepare a large pot with boiling water. I usually pre-boil the water before putting it in the pot and then set the burner to achieve a rapid boil when I am at step 8
2. Prepare your workspace with parchment
3. Put on nitrile gloves (important when using fruit or vegetable powders as they will stain!)
4. In a medium mixing bowl, blend together all dry ingredients (minus the ¼ C arrowroot used in the final kneading)
5. In a small ramekin, beat together egg yolks and full egg
6. Make a well in the center of the dry ingredients and pour egg the egg mixture in the center of the well
7. Using a fork, gradually blend in flour mixture into beaten eggs. (Picture drawing in the flour from the edges and working it into the eggs on a gradual yet continual basis)
8. When you cannot use your fork anymore, begin hand mixing and kneading of the pasta dough for five minutes
9. At the end of five minutes scatter the ¼ C arrowroot on your parchment and place dough on top of loose arrowroot. Knead additional arrowroot into the dough to achieve the texture discussed in Chapter Two.

At this point either roll to 1/8 inch on your already floured parchment paper by using a top sheet of parchment between your rolling pin and dough and slicing by hand or a pastry cutter, using a hand-crank roller and slicer, or use an automated roller and slicer. Once you have your sliced pasta, immediately toss it into rapidly boiling water for 5 minutes or until done to your particular texture tastes. Unlike conventional pasta you'd find in the grocery store, and even some gluten-free pastas, I've not found the basic recipe go to "mush" from overcooking.

Beet Pasta

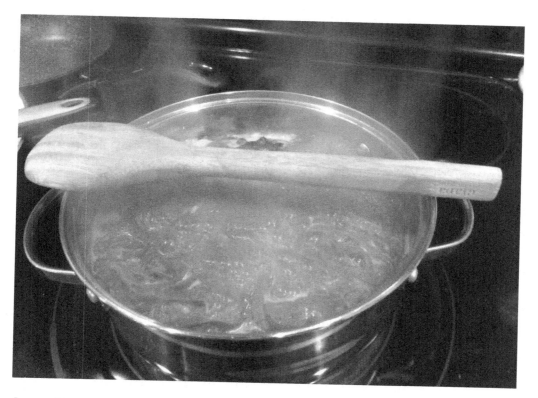

Ingredients:
- ½ C Ultra-fine ground almond flour
- 1/3 C Tapioca flour
- 1/3 C Arrowroot flour + ¼ C for final kneading
- 2-3 T Beet powder
- 2 t Himalayan salt
- 2 Large egg yolks
- 1 Large egg

Instructions:

1. Prepare a large pot with boiling water. I usually pre-boil the water before putting it in the pot and then set the burner to achieve a rapid boil when I am at step 8
2. Prepare your workspace with parchment
3. Put on nitrile gloves (important when using fruit or vegetable powders as they will stain!)
4. In a medium mixing bowl, blend together all dry ingredients (minus the ¼ C arrowroot used in the final kneading)
5. In a small ramekin, beat together egg yolks and full egg
6. Make a well in the center of the dry ingredients and pour egg the egg mixture in the center of the well
7. Using a fork, gradually blend in flour mixture into beaten eggs. (Picture drawing in the flour from the edges and working it into the eggs on a gradual yet continual basis)
8. When you cannot use your fork anymore, begin hand mixing and kneading of the pasta dough for five minutes
9. At the end of five minutes scatter the ¼ C arrowroot on your parchment and place dough on top of loose arrowroot. Knead additional arrowroot into the dough to achieve the texture discussed in Chapter Two.

At this point either roll to 1/8 inch on your already floured parchment paper by using a top sheet of parchment between your rolling pin and dough and slicing by hand or a pastry cutter, using a hand-crank roller and slicer, or use an automated roller and slicer. Once you have your sliced pasta, immediately toss it into rapidly boiling water for 5 minutes or until done to your particular texture tastes. Unlike conventional pasta you'd find in the grocery store, and even some gluten-free pastas, I've not found the basic recipe go to "mush" from overcooking.

Strawberry Pasta

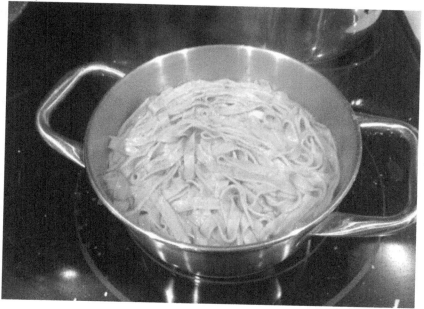

This is another example where you'll notice the difference in color when making your Paleo pasta between the before/raw state and much lighter color of the cooked. It's natural, all part of the boiling process, you didn't do anything wrong, and it won't lose a bit of flavor!

Ingredients:

- ½ C Ultra-fine ground almond flour
- 1/2 C Tapioca flour
- 1/3 C Arrowroot flour + ¼ C for final kneading
- 2 T Strawberry powder
- 1 t Himalayan salt
- 2 Large egg yolks
- 1 Large egg

Instructions:

1. Prepare a large pot with boiling water. I usually pre-boil the water before putting it in the pot and then set the burner to achieve a rapid boil when I am at step 8
2. Prepare your workspace with parchment
3. Put on nitrile gloves (important when using fruit or vegetable powders as they will stain!)
4. In a medium mixing bowl, blend together all dry ingredients (minus the ¼ C arrowroot used in the final kneading)
5. In a small ramekin, beat together egg yolks and full egg
6. Make a well in the center of the dry ingredients and pour egg the egg mixture in the center of the well
7. Using a fork, gradually blend in flour mixture into beaten eggs. (Picture drawing in the flour from the edges and working it into the eggs on a gradual yet continual basis)
8. When you cannot use your fork anymore, begin hand mixing and kneading of the pasta dough for five minutes
9. At the end of five minutes scatter the ¼ C arrowroot on your parchment and place dough on top of loose arrowroot. Knead additional arrowroot into the dough to achieve the texture discussed in Chapter Two.

At this point either roll to 1/8 inch on your already floured parchment paper by using a top sheet of parchment between your rolling pin and dough and slicing by hand or a pastry cutter, using a hand-crank roller and slicer, or use an automated roller and slicer. Once you have your sliced pasta, immediately toss it into rapidly boiling water for 5 minutes or until done to your particular texture tastes. Unlike conventional pasta you'd find in the grocery store, and even some gluten-free pastas, I've not found the basic recipe go to "mush" from overcooking.

Banana Flour Pasta
Ingredients:

- ½ C Banana flour
- ½ C Ultra-fine ground almond flour
- 1/4 C Tapioca flour
- 1/4 C Arrowroot flour + ¼ C for final kneading
- 2 T Powdered agave nectar or Swerve
- 2 Large egg yolks
- 1 Large egg

Instructions:

1. Prepare a large pot with boiling water. I usually pre-boil the water before putting it in the pot and then set the burner to achieve a rapid boil when I am at step 8
2. Prepare your workspace with parchment
3. Put on nitrile gloves (important when using fruit or vegetable powders as they will stain!)
4. In a medium mixing bowl, blend together all dry ingredients (minus the ¼ C arrowroot used in the final kneading)
5. In a small ramekin, beat together egg yolks and full egg
6. Make a well in the center of the dry ingredients and pour egg the egg mixture in the center of the well
7. Using a fork, gradually blend in flour mixture into beaten eggs. (Picture drawing in the flour from the edges and working it into the eggs on a gradual yet continual basis)
8. When you cannot use your fork anymore, begin hand mixing and kneading of the pasta dough for five minutes
9. At the end of five minutes scatter the ¼ C arrowroot on your parchment and place dough on top of loose arrowroot. Knead additional arrowroot into the dough to achieve the texture discussed in Chapter Two.

At this point either roll to 1/8 inch on your already floured parchment paper by using a top sheet of parchment between your rolling pin and dough and slicing by hand or a pastry cutter, using a hand-crank roller and slicer, or use an automated roller and slicer. Once you have your sliced pasta, immediately toss it into rapidly boiling water for 10 minutes or until done to your particular texture tastes. Banana flour pasta is a bit heartier, so it takes longer to cook than the basic pasta recipe.

NOTE: In lieu of powdered agave, do not be tempted to use regular liquid agave. The dough will end up being a sticky mess or overly starchy and will not roll or cook properly.

Merlot Flour Pasta

Ingredients:

- ½ C Ultra-fine ground almond flour
- 1/2 C Tapioca flour
- 1/3 C Arrowroot flour + ¼ C for final kneading
- 2 T Merlot grape skin flour
- 1 t Himalayan salt
- 2 Large egg yolks
- 1 Large egg
- 1 t Spring water (if necessary)

Instructions:

1. Prepare a large pot with boiling water. I usually pre-boil the water before putting it in the pot and then set the burner to achieve a rapid boil when I am at step 8
2. Prepare your workspace with parchment
3. Put on nitrile gloves (important when using fruit or vegetable powders as they will stain!)
4. In a medium mixing bowl, blend together all dry ingredients (minus the ¼ C arrowroot used in the final kneading)
5. In a small ramekin, beat together egg yolks and full egg
6. Make a well in the center of the dry ingredients and pour egg the egg mixture in the center of the well
7. Using a fork, gradually blend in flour mixture into beaten eggs. (Picture drawing in the flour from the edges and working it into the eggs on a gradual yet continual basis)
8. When you cannot use your fork anymore, begin hand mixing and kneading of the pasta dough for five minutes. If the dough is too dry and crumbly, add water ¼ t at a time and continue to knead until the right texture is achieved

9. At the end of five minutes scatter the ¼ C arrowroot on your parchment and place dough on top of loose arrowroot. Knead additional arrowroot into the dough to achieve the texture discussed in Chapter Two.

At this point either roll to 1/8 inch on your already floured parchment paper by using a top sheet of parchment between your rolling pin and dough and slicing by hand or a pastry cutter, using a hand-crank roller and slicer, or use an automated roller and slicer. Once you have your sliced pasta, immediately toss it into rapidly boiling water for 5 minutes or until done to your particular texture tastes. Unlike conventional pasta you'd find in the grocery store, and even some gluten-free pastas, I've not found the basic recipe go to "mush" from overcooking.

NOTE: Like many of the unique flours highlighted throughout this chapter, wine grape skin is HIGHLY absorbent, much like coconut flour.

Chardonnay Flour Pasta

Ingredients:

- ½ C Ultra-fine ground almond flour
- 1/2 C Tapioca flour
- 1/3 C Arrowroot flour + ¼ C for final kneading
- 2 T Merlot grape skin flour
- 1 t Himalayan salt
- 2 Large egg yolks
- 1 Large egg
- 1 t Spring water (if necessary)

Instructions:

1. Prepare a large pot with boiling water. I usually pre-boil the water before putting it in the pot and then set the burner to achieve a rapid boil when I am at step 8
2. Prepare your workspace with parchment
3. Put on nitrile gloves (important when using fruit or vegetable powders as they will stain!)
4. In a medium mixing bowl, blend together all dry ingredients (minus the ¼ C arrowroot used in the final kneading)
5. In a small ramekin, beat together egg yolks and full egg
6. Make a well in the center of the dry ingredients and pour egg the egg mixture in the center of the well
7. Using a fork, gradually blend in flour mixture into beaten eggs. (Picture drawing in the flour from the edges and working it into the eggs on a gradual yet continual basis)
8. When you cannot use your fork anymore, begin hand mixing and kneading of the pasta dough for five minutes. If the dough is too dry and crumbly, add water ¼ t at a time and continue to knead until the right texture is achieved

9. At the end of five minutes scatter the ¼ C arrowroot on your parchment and place dough on top of loose arrowroot. Knead additional arrowroot into the dough to achieve the texture discussed in Chapter Two.

At this point either roll to 1/8 inch on your already floured parchment paper by using a top sheet of parchment between your rolling pin and dough and slicing by hand or a pastry cutter, using a hand-crank roller and slicer, or use an automated roller and slicer. Once you have your sliced pasta, immediately toss it into rapidly boiling water for 5 minutes or until done to your particular texture tastes. Unlike conventional pasta you'd find in the grocery store, and even some gluten-free pastas, I've not found the basic recipe go to "mush" from overcooking.

NOTE: Like many of the unique flours highlighted throughout this chapter, wine grape skin is HIGHLY absorbent, much like coconut flour.

Butternut Squash Pasta

Ingredients:

- ½ C Ultra-fine ground almond flour
- 1/2 C Tapioca flour
- 1/3 C Arrowroot flour + ¼ C for final kneading
- 1 T Butternut squash puree
- 1 t Himalayan salt
- 1 Large egg yolk
- 1 Large egg

Instructions:

1. Prepare a large pot with boiling water. I usually pre-boil the water before putting it in the pot and then set the burner to achieve a rapid boil when I am at step 8
2. Prepare your workspace with parchment
3. Put on nitrile gloves (important when using fruit or vegetable powders as they will stain!)
4. In a medium mixing bowl, blend together all dry ingredients (minus the ¼ C arrowroot used in the final kneading)
5. In a small ramekin, beat together butternut squash puree, egg yolk, and full egg
6. Make a well in the center of the dry ingredients and pour egg the egg mixture in the center of the well
7. Using a fork, gradually blend in flour mixture into beaten eggs. (Picture drawing in the flour from the edges and working it into the eggs on a gradual yet continual basis)
8. When you cannot use your fork anymore, begin hand mixing and kneading of the pasta dough for five minutes. If the dough is too dry and crumbly, add water ¼ t at a time and continue to knead until the right texture is achieved

9. At the end of five minutes scatter the ¼ C arrowroot on your parchment and place dough on top of loose arrowroot. Knead additional arrowroot into the dough to achieve the texture discussed in Chapter Two.

At this point either roll to 1/8 inch on your already floured parchment paper by using a top sheet of parchment between your rolling pin and dough and slicing by hand or a pastry cutter, using a hand-crank roller and slicer, or use an automated roller and slicer. Once you have your sliced pasta, immediately toss it into rapidly boiling water for 5 minutes or until done to your particular texture tastes. Unlike conventional pasta you'd find in the grocery store, and even some gluten-free pastas, I've not found the basic recipe go to "mush" from overcooking.

Chocolate Pasta

Ingredients:

- ¼ C + 1 T Dutch cocoa flour (or other cocoa powder)
- ½ C Ultra-fine ground almond flour
- ¼ + ¼ C Arrowroot flour
- ½ t Himalayan sea salt
- 2 Large egg yolks
- 1 Large egg
- 1 T Vanilla powder
- 3 T Powdered agave nectar

Instructions:

1. Prepare a large pot with boiling water. I usually pre-boil the water before putting it in the pot and then set the burner to achieve a rapid boil when I am at step 8
2. Prepare your workspace with parchment
3. Put on nitrile gloves
4. In a medium mixing bowl, blend together all dry ingredients (minus the additional ¼ C arrowroot used in the final kneading)
5. In a small ramekin, beat together egg yolks and full egg
6. Make a well in the center of the dry ingredients and pour egg the egg mixture in the center of the well
7. Using a fork, gradually blend in flour mixture into beaten eggs. (Picture drawing in the flour from the edges and working it into the eggs on a gradual yet continual basis)
8. When you cannot use your fork anymore, begin hand mixing and kneading of the pasta dough for five minutes
9. At the end of five minutes scatter the ¼ C arrowroot on your parchment and place dough on top of loose arrowroot. Knead additional arrowroot into the dough to achieve the texture discussed in Chapter Two.

At this point either roll to 1/8 inch on your already floured parchment paper by using a top sheet of parchment between your rolling pin and dough and slicing by hand or a pastry cutter. Once you have your sliced pasta, immediately toss it into rapidly boiling water for 5 minutes or until done to your particular texture tastes. Unlike conventional pasta you'd find in the grocery store, and even some gluten-free pastas, I've not found the basic recipe go to "mush" from overcooking.

Coffee Flour Pasta

Ingredients:

- ½ C Coffee flour
- ½ C Ultra-fine ground almond flour
- ¼ C Arrowroot flour
- 2 t Himalayan sea salt
- 2 Large egg yolks
- 1 Large egg
- 3 T Powdered agave nectar
- 2 T Espresso

Instructions:

1. Prepare a large pot with boiling water. I usually pre-boil the water before putting it in the pot and then set the burner to achieve a rapid boil when I am at step 8
2. Prepare your workspace with parchment
3. Put on nitrile gloves (important when using coffee flour as it will stain!)
4. In a medium mixing bowl, blend together all dry ingredients (minus the ¼ C arrowroot used in the final kneading)
5. In a small ramekin, beat together egg yolks and full egg
6. Make a well in the center of the dry ingredients and pour egg the egg mixture in the center of the well
7. Using a fork, gradually blend in flour mixture into beaten eggs. (Picture drawing in the flour from the edges and working it into the eggs on a gradual yet continual basis)
8. When you cannot use your fork anymore, begin hand mixing and kneading of the pasta dough for five minutes
9. At the end of five minutes scatter the ¼ C arrowroot on your parchment and place dough on top of loose arrowroot. Knead additional arrowroot into the dough to achieve the texture discussed in Chapter Two.

At this point either roll to 1/8 inch on your already floured parchment paper by using a top sheet of parchment between your rolling pin and dough and slicing by hand or a pastry cutter. Once you have your sliced pasta, immediately toss it into rapidly boiling water for 5 minutes or until done to your particular texture tastes. Unlike conventional pasta you'd find in the grocery store, and even some gluten-free pastas, I've not found the basic recipe go to "mush" from overcooking.

NOTE: Coffee flour is a unique baking medium; it maintains a slightly gritty texture even after baking or cooking. It also absorbs water much like coconut flour; thus, you'll have to play around a bit with the amount of espresso you end up using; literally drizzling in any additional moisture to get the dough you're looking for.

It might be because of the gritty texture, but, I recommend rolling this out by hand on parchment and using a pastry cutter or knife to slice the dough before boiling. It does not roll well in automated rollers.

Lemon Pasta
- ½ C Ultra-fine ground almond flour
- 1/3 C Tapioca flour
- 1/3 C Arrowroot flour + ¼ C for final kneading
- 5 – 10 drops of Lemon oil, depending on the strength of the taste you desire
- 2 t Himalayan salt
- 2 Large egg yolks
- 1 Large egg

Instructions:

1. Prepare a large pot with boiling water. I usually pre-boil the water before putting it in the pot and then set the burner to achieve a rapid boil when I am at step 8
2. Prepare your workspace with parchment
3. Put on nitrile gloves
4. In a medium mixing bowl, blend together all dry ingredients (minus the ¼ C arrowroot used in the final kneading)
5. In a small ramekin, beat together egg yolks and full egg
6. Make a well in the center of the dry ingredients and pour egg the egg mixture in the center of the well
7. Using a fork, gradually blend in flour mixture into beaten eggs. (Picture drawing in the flour from the edges and working it into the eggs on a gradual yet continual basis)
8. When you cannot use your fork anymore, begin hand mixing and kneading of the pasta dough for five minutes
9. At the end of five minutes scatter the ¼ C arrowroot on your parchment and place dough on top of loose arrowroot. Knead additional arrowroot into the dough to achieve the texture discussed in Chapter Two.

At this point either roll to 1/8 inch on your already floured parchment paper by using a top sheet of parchment between your rolling pin and dough and slicing by hand or a pastry cutter, using a hand-crank roller and slicer, or use an automated roller and slicer. Once you have your sliced pasta, immediately toss it into rapidly boiling water for 5 minutes or until done to your particular texture tastes. Unlike conventional pasta you'd find in the grocery store, and even some gluten-free pastas, I've not found the basic recipe go to "mush" from overcooking.

Chapter Six: Sauces and More

Pesto Sauce
Ingredients:

- 2 C Fresh basil leaves
- 1/4 C Almonds
- 2 t Nutritional yeast flakes
- 2 t Minced garlic
- ½ t Himalayan sea salt
- ½ C Mediterranean olive oil
- ¼ C Avocado mayonnaise

Instructions:

1. Place fresh basil, almonds, nutritional yeast, garlic, and salt in a food process and process on high for about 30 seconds to create a paste. You may have to scrape down sides and process again.
2. Add olive oil and process again until all ingredients are well combined
3. Add avocado mayonnaise and pulse to incorporate into a creamy sauce.
4. Can be stored in the refrigerator for up to a week.

Ricotta Cheese

Ingredients:

- 1½ C Raw cashews, cooked
- 1 t Lemon zest
- 3 T Lemon juice
- 1 t Minced garlic
- ¼ C Unsweetened almond/coconut milk (any Paleo nut milk is fine)
- ¼ C Spring water (use as needed to achieve your desired consistency)

Instructions:

1. Blend all ingredients together in a high-speed blender. You may need to scrape down the sides frequently.

NOTE: To cook, raw cashews can either be soaked overnight or boiled for 30 minutes, completely cooled, and rinsed thoroughly.

Cheddar Cheese

Ingredients:

- 1½ C Water
- 2 T Unflavored gelatin
- ½ C Raw cashews, cooked
- ¼ C Nutritional yeast flakes
- 3 T Fresh lemon juice
- 2 T Sesame tahini
- 3 t Smoked paprika (sweet or hot depending on your desired flavor profile)
- 3 t Onion powder
- 1½ t Himalayan sea salt
- ½ t Garlic powder
- ¼ t Dry mustard powder

Instructions:

1. Grease a one-quart sized glass bowl with coconut oil and set aside.
2. Place prepared cashews, nutritional yeast flakes, lemon juice, tahini, and all seasonings in a tall cylindrical carafe (I use the carafe from a 32 oz. French press).
3. Once all other ingredients are in the blender, bring gelatin and water to a rapid boil for 1 minute and immediately pour the hot gelatin mixture into your blender and blend on the highest speed until the "unset" cheese is a very smooth texture. It should not be grainy at all. Ideally, you want this almost the consistency of a thick, but not quite Greek yogurt thick.
4. Once you've achieved the proper consistency, pour your cheese mixture into the prepared bowl and place in the refrigerator for a minimum of three hours, uncovered. After three hours, cover with saran wrap overnight before use.

NOTE: To cook, raw cashews can either be soaked overnight or boiled for 30 minutes, completely cooled, and rinsed thoroughly.

Alfredo Sauce

Ingredients:

- 2 C Raw cashews, cooked
- 2 C Unsweetened almond/coconut milk
- 2 t Lemon juice
- 8-10 cloves Fresh garlic
- 2 T + 1 t Mediterranean olive oil
- 2 T Ghee
- 1 t Himalayan sea salt
- ¼ t Ground peppercorn to taste

Instructions:

1. Preheat oven to 350 degrees
2. Cut off the top of garlic head, and using a pastry brush, liberally brush the oil with about 1 teaspoon olive oil
3. Wrap garlic head in aluminum foil, place on a baking pan with a lip, and bake 45 minutes
4. Sauté onions in 1 teaspoon of olive oil until onions become translucent
5. Remove garlic from oven, and carefully unwrap. The garlic cloves should easily squeeze out of the head. Squeeze all into a food processor
6. Add onions and pulse together
7. Add all other remaining ingredients into food processor and process until smooth and creamy
8. Use immediately or refrigerate in an airtight jar or can according to your canning directions

NOTE: To cook, raw cashews can either be soaked overnight or boiled for 30 minutes, completely cooled, and rinsed thoroughly. Also, instead of a blender, you can use a food processor, but it will not turn out as creamy and smooth, and the sauce will have a slightly gritty texture.

Lobster Cream Sauce

Ingredients:

- 2 4 oz. Lobster tails, steamed and diced
- 1 C Coconut cream
- 1 T Lemon juice
- 2 T Ghee or butter from grass-fed cows
- 1 t Minced garlic
- Himalayan Sea salt and black pepper to taste
- 2 t Tapioca flour
- 2 t Spring water, cold

Instructions:

1. In a large skillet over medium heat, melt ghee or butter
2. Add garlic and cook for 1 – 2 minutes
3. While garlic is cooking make your slurry: combine tapioca flour and water in a small ramekin and stir well to dissolve all tapioca flour assuring no lumps. For this step, the water must be COLD
4. Add lemon juice to garlic in skillet and stir to incorporate all ingredients
5. Whisk in coconut cream
6. Slowly add your slurry to the skillet, continuing to whisk all ingredients together as the slurry is being poured in
7. Continue to stir until sauce is the thickness you desire and then immediately remove from heat
8. Fold in your diced lobster with a wooden spoon.

Mushroom Cream Sauce

Ingredients:

- 2 T Ghee or butter from grass-fed cows
- 2 t Minced garlic
- ½ t Sage
- Himalayan sea salt and pepper, to taste
- 10 oz. Baby Bella mushroom caps, finely diced
- 2 t Tapioca flour
- 2 t Spring water, cold
- 1 C Coconut cream

Instructions:

1. In a large skillet over medium heat, melt ghee or butter
2. Add garlic and cook for 1 – 2 minutes
3. While garlic is cooking make your slurry: combine tapioca flour and water in a small ramekin and stir well to dissolve all tapioca flour assuring no lumps. For this step, the water must be COLD
4. Add diced mushrooms and cook for approximately 5 – 8 minutes or until mushrooms are well done and tender
5. Whisk in coconut cream
6. Slowly add your slurry to the skillet, continuing to whisk all ingredients together as the slurry is being poured in
7. Continue to stir until sauce is the thickness you desire and then immediately remove from heat.

Lemon Cashew Sauce

Ingredients:

- 1 ½ C Raw cashews, cooked
- ½ C Unsweetened almond/coconut milk
- ½ C Lemon juice
- 2 t Lemon zest
- 2 T Nutritional yeast flakes
- 1 t Himalayan sea salt

Instructions:

1. Combine all ingredients in a high-speed blender and process until smooth and creamy
2. Use immediately or refrigerate in an airtight jar or can according to your canning directions.

NOTE: To cook, raw cashews can either be soaked overnight or boiled for 30 minutes, completely cooled, and rinsed thoroughly. Also, instead of a blender, you can use a food processor, but it will not turn out as creamy and smooth, and the sauce will have a slightly gritty texture.

Marinara Sauce

Ingredients:

- 28 oz. can Peeled tomatoes (with no additives)
- 15 oz. can Tomato sauce (with no additives)
- ½ Yellow onion, diced
- 2 T Mediterranean olive oil
- 2 t Minced garlic
- 1 t Coconut garlic sauce
- 2 t Oregano
- 2 t Basil
- Himalayan sea salt & pepper to taste

Instructions:

1. In a large saucepan over medium heat, sauté onion in olive oil for about 5 minutes
2. Add garlic and sauté together for an additional minute
3. Add remaining ingredients
4. Heat on medium to a soft boil, reduce heat, and simmer for 20 minutes
5. Allow to cool and refrigerate in an airtight jar

Pine Nut, Mushroom and Walnut Cream Sauce
Ingredients:

- 2 T Mediterranean olive oil
- 2 T Minced garlic
- ½ Yellow onion, chopped finely
- 10 oz. Baby Bella mushrooms, finely diced
- 1 C Coconut cream
- 2 T Nutritional yeast flakes
- ½ C Pine nuts, toasted
- ½ C Blanched walnuts, chopped
- 2 t Tapioca flour
- 2 t Spring water (cold)

Instructions:

1. Preheat oven 325
2. On a parchment lined baking pan, spread out pine nuts
3. Once oven comes to temperature, cook pine nuts for 8 minutes, or just until fragrant, stirring half way through to avoid burning.
4. Remove pine nuts from oven and allow to cool.
5. While pine nuts are toasting, stir tapioca flour and cold water in a ramekin to completely dissolve the tapioca and assure there are no lumps; set aside
6. In a large skillet heat olive oil over medium heat
7. Add garlic and onion and cook until onion is translucent
8. Add mushrooms and cook a further 5 minutes or until just tender
9. Whisk in coconut cream, nutritional yeast flakes, pine nuts, and walnuts, simmering sauce until completely heated
10. Gradually whisk in tapioca/water slurry until desired sauce thinness is achieved and remove from heat.

Basic Vodka Sauce

Ingredients:

- ½ Ghee or butter from grass-fed cows
- ½ Yellow onion, finely diced
- 1 C Vodka (make certain your Vodka is Paleo-friendly; you can get grain-free vodka made from potatoes)
- 1 large can Fire-roasted crushed tomatoes
- 1 can Coconut cream (approximately 15oz.)

Instructions:

1. In a large skillet over medium heat, sauté onion in ghee or butter until slightly brown and soft, approximately 8 – 10 minutes
2. Pour in vodka and let cook/reduce for 10 minutes
3. Mix in crushed tomatoes, reduce heat to simmer and cook for 30 minutes
4. Whisk in coconut cream and simmer for another 30 minutes

Tomato Cream Sauce

Ingredients:

- ½ Ghee or butter from grass-fed cows
- ½ Yellow onion, finely diced
- 1 large can Fire-roasted crushed tomatoes
- 1 can Coconut cream (approximately 15oz)

Instructions:

1. In a large skillet over medium heat, sauté onion in ghee or butter until slightly brown and soft, approximately 8 – 10 minutes
2. Mix in crushed tomatoes, reduce heat to simmer and cook for 30 minutes
3. Whisk in coconut cream and simmer for another 30 minutes.

Garlic Basil Sauce

Ingredients:

- ½ Yellow onion, finely diced
- 1 T Minced garlic
- ¼ C Mediterranean olive oil
- 1 large can Fire-roasted crushed tomatoes
- 15 fresh Basil leaves, finely chopped or 2 T dried basil
- 3 T Fresh parsley, finely chopped
- 1 t Himalayan sea salt
- ½ t Black pepper, coarse ground

Instructions:

1. Pour olive oil into a Dutch oven, bringing to heat over medium setting
2. Once oil is hot, sauté onion and garlic in oil until tender, approximately 8 minutes
3. Add remaining ingredients and bring to a boil
4. Immediately reduce heat to low
5. Cover and simmer for one to two hours.

Chapter Seven: Pasta Main Meals

Spaghetti

Ingredients:

- 1 batch Basic Paleo Pasta recipe (optional tomato or spinach Paleo pasta)
- 1 lb. Ground sirloin from grass-fed cows (optional lean ground turkey)
- 1 large can Fire roasted crushed tomatoes
- 3 T Mediterranean olive oil
- 1 T Fresh basil
- 2 t Minced garlic
- ½ Yellow onion, diced
- 10 oz. Baby Bella mushrooms, sliced
- 1 T Coconut garlic sauce
- ½ t Himalayan sea salt

Instructions:

1. In a large pan, add olive oil
2. Add sliced mushrooms, diced onion, and garlic and sauté until tender and onions are translucent
3. Remove vegetables from pan with a slotted spoon
4. Add ground beef to pan, and brown
5. When ground beef is browned, add sautéed vegetables, crushed tomatoes and spices, mixing to incorporate all.
6. Bring to a light boil, then turn down heat to simmer until Paleo Pasta is complete.
7. Begin your Paleo Pasta of choice using a spaghetti disk or cutter, or slice very thin like spaghetti if manually cutting the pasta!

NOTE: Use spaghetti disk if using a fully automated pasta machine. Also, make spaghetti sauce first – it always gets better the longer it simmers and flavors have a chance to blend.

Beef Lasagna
Ingredients:
- 1 batch of Spaghetti sauce
- 12 oz. Paleo ricotta cheese (recipe in this book)
- 1 batch of Basic Paleo Pasta (spinach or tomato pasta optional)
- 24 Fresh basil leaves

Instructions:
1. Pre-heat oven to 375 degrees
2. Make spaghetti sauce and allow to cool slightly
3. Make Paleo pasta "flavor" of your choice. In this case, strictly roll the dough if making your pasta manually, or with rollers if using a pasta maker. You want strips of dough
4. Cook your pasta dough strips and cool completely to allow for handling without getting burned
5. In a lasagna pan, ladle a small amount of spaghetti sauce in the bottom of the pan
6. Begin the layering process: layer strips of pasta followed by additional spaghetti sauce, then small dollops of Paleo ricotta cheese (ideally, spread them together once placed in the pan with the back of a spoon or knife), then top with 12 fresh basil leaves. Repeat the process until your lasagna is complete.
7. Place in oven and bake for 45 minutes

NOTE: Slice Paleo pasta into 2" strips if manually rolling, using the lasagna disk in an automatic pasta machine, or use directly from the pasta rolling/flattening device.

Vegetable Lasagna

Ingredients:
- 1 batch of Spaghetti sauce made without ground sirloin
- 1 medium Zucchini, thinly sliced
- 12 oz. Paleo ricotta cheese (recipe in this book)
- 1 batch of Basic Paleo Pasta (spinach or tomato pasta optional)
- 24 Fresh Basil leaves

Instructions:
1. Pre-heat oven to 375 degrees
2. Make spaghetti sauce, substituting zucchini slices for ground beef, and allow to cool slightly
3. Make Paleo pasta "flavor" of your choice. In this case, strictly roll the dough if making your pasta manually, or with rollers if using a pasta maker. You want strips of dough
4. Cook your pasta dough strips and cool completely to allow for handling without getting burned
5. In a lasagna pan, ladle a small amount of spaghetti sauce in the bottom of the pan
6. Begin the layering process: layer strips of pasta followed by additional spaghetti sauce, then small dollops of Paleo ricotta cheese (ideally, spread them together once placed in the pan with the back of a spoon or knife), then top with 12 fresh basil leaves. Repeat the process until your lasagna is complete.
7. Place in oven and bake for 45 minutes

NOTE: Slice Paleo pasta into 2" strips if manually rolling, using the lasagna disk in an automatic pasta machine, or use directly from the pasta rolling/flattening device.

Pesto Chicken

Ingredients:

- 1 batch Basic or lemon pasta
- 1 batch Pesto sauce
- 3 Chicken breasts, diced
- 2 T Mediterranean olive oil

Instructions:

1. In a large skillet heat the olive oil over medium heat. Add the diced chicken and cook thoroughly until insides of diced pieces are no longer pink
2. Add the pesto sauce, stir well, and continue heating over medium heat setting.
3. Add the basic or lemon pasta and gently mix with a wooden spoon to distribute pesto sauce throughout
4. Once heated, enjoy!

Taco Pasta

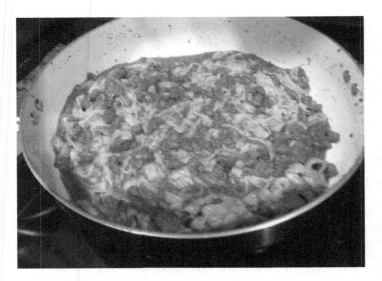

Ingredients:
- 3 T Mediterranean olive oil
- 2 T Tapioca flour
- 2 T Water, cold
- 1 lb. Grass-fed ground beef
- 3 t Sweet paprika
- 1 t Ground onion
- 1 t Ground garlic
- 1 t Chili powder
- 1 t Oregano
- 1 batch Basic pasta

Instructions:
1. In a large skillet heat the olive oil over medium heat. Add the ground beef and cook thoroughly

2. While beef is browning, make your slurry. Combine tapioca flour and cold water, stirring well to dissolve four and assure there are no lumps
3. Add spices and stir until meat is well coated
4. Add ¾ C water, stir well, and bring to a boil
5. Add slurry and stir continually as sauce thickens
6. Once sauce is to desired thickness remove from heat immediately
7. Add the basic pasta and gently mix with a wooden spoon to distribute taco sauce throughout
8. Once heated, enjoy!

Goulash
Ingredients:
- 3 T Mediterranean olive oil
- 1 lb. Ground Beef
- ½ t Himalayan sea salt
- Black Pepper to taste
- 2 t Minced garlic
- ½ Yellow onion, finely diced
- 1 large can Fire-roasted diced or crushed tomatoes
- 2 T Coconut aminos
- 3 T Tomato paste
- ½ C Spring water
- ½ t Caraway seeds
- ½ t Thyme
- 1 T Hungarian paprika
- 2 T Tapioca flour
- 2 T Spring water, cold

Instructions:
1. Brown ground beef in a large skillet over medium heat in olive oil
2. As meat is browning, add salt and pepper to taste
3. As meat is browning, make your slurry from tapioca flour and water, stirring completely to dissolve and make sure there are no lumps
4. When meat is almost completely cooked, add garlic and onion, stirring frequently for about 3 minutes
5. Add tomatoes, coconut aminos, tomato paste, and water and bring to a boil
6. Reduce heat to simmer and add Stir in the caraway, thyme, and paprika, cooking on simmer for about 20 minutes

7. If sauce is too thin, add slurry and stir until sauce is to desired consistency then immediately remove from heat
8. Add pasta and gently stir with a wooden spoon to combine

NOTE: for purposes of this dish, if you are using an automatic pasta machine you may wish to use a macaroni disk; otherwise fettuccini cut works well.

Mock Beef Stroganoff

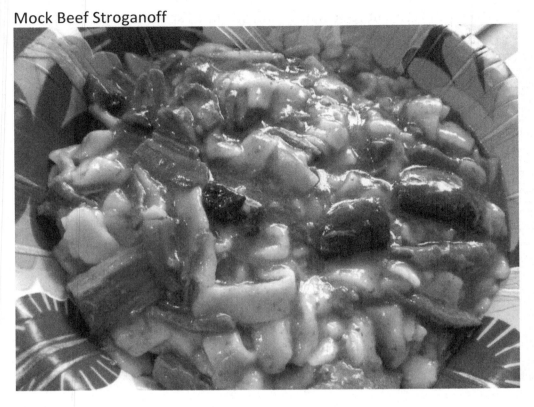

Ingredients:

- 1 T + 3T   Mediterranean Olive Oil
- ½ Yellow onion, finely diced
- 10oz. Baby Bella mushrooms, roughly chopped
- 3 t Minced garlic
- ½ t Himalayan Sea salt
- ½ t Black pepper, coarsely ground (to taste)
- 1 C Organic Paleo vegetable broth
- 1 C Full fat coconut milk, or almond/coconut milk bend
- 1.5 lbs. Grass-fed sirloin tip roast cut into small pieces or grass-fed stew meat cutting beef chunks into smaller pieces
- 1 batch Basic Paleo pasta
- Paleo sour cream (optional)

Instructions:

1. Add 1 T olive oil to a heavy soup pot over medium heat, then add onions, mushrooms and a pinch of salt
2. Sauté for 10-12 minutes or until onions are translucent and mushrooms are soft
3. Add garlic and spices, stirring in the spices to integrate with vegetables
4. Add vegetable broth and coconut or coconut/almond milk
5. Let the mixture simmer for about 10 minutes
6. Blend with an immersion blender
7. If the soup is not thick enough, add 2 t tapioca flour mixed with 2 t COLD water to create a slurry, stirring continually until desired thickness of a sauce is achieved then remove from heat immediately and set aside
8. Heat a large skillet over medium heat and add remaining 3 T Mediterranean Olive Oil
9. When oil is heated, add beef chunks and brown (more cooking than searing) while stirring to prevent burning
10. When beef appears thoroughly cooked, add mushroom caps and sauté the entire mixture until mushroom caps appear tender
11. Add cream of mushroom base mixture and cook for 30 minutes on low heat to bring flavors together
12. Add basic Paleo pasta and serve with Paleo sour cream if desired

Mock Beef Bourguignon with Merlot Pasta

Ingredients:

- 2 t Extra Virgin olive oil
- 3 Slices Paleo bacon, chopped
- 3 T Ghee or butter from the milk of grass fed cows
- 10 oz. White mushrooms, medium in size, wiped with damp cloth to clean, thinly sliced
- ½ t Himalayan sea salt
- ½ t Ground black pepper, coarsely ground (or to taste)
- 1 C Pearl onions
- 1.5 lbs. Grass-fed tri-top roast or grass-fed stew meat
- 3 T Tapioca flour
- 3 C Beef bone broth
- Bouquet of 3 or 4 sprigs each sage and fresh thyme, tied with kitchen string
- 1 batch Merlot pasta

Instructions:

1. Heat a large deep skillet
2. When heated, add olive oil
3. When olive oil is heated, add bacon to the pan and brown
4. When bacon is nicely browned, remove cooked bacon from pan and set aside
5. Add half the ghee (1 ½ T) and melt into the bacon drippings still in the pan
6. Add mushrooms to the pan and turn to coat evenly with ghee/butter and bacon grease, sauté mushrooms 2 to 3 minutes
7. Add onions to the mushrooms and cook an additional 3 minutes
8. Remove mushrooms and onions onto a temporary holding plate using a slotted spoon

9. Add remaining 1 ½ T ghee to the pan and melt it, then add meat to the very hot pan and brown evenly on all sides, being careful not to burn or scorch the meat
10. Add tapioca flour to browned meat in the pan and cook an additional 2 minutes.
11. Add 1 C beef bone broth to the pan slowly while stirring
12. Bring to a boil and deglaze pan while stirring
13. Once pan is deglazed, add remaining bone broth and spice packet
14. Cover pan and bring to a boil
15. Once the beef dish is boiling, reduce heat to medium and continue to cook and additional five minutes while still covered
16. After mixture has cooked for five minutes, add onions, mushrooms, and bacon back into the pot and cook without the lid until sauce thickens
13. If sauce is not thick enough, you can always add 2 t tapioca flour mixed with 2 t COLD water to create a slurry, stirring continually until desired thickness of a sauce is achieved then remove from heat immediately and set aside
14. Once sauce is thickened, add hot Merlot Pasta and stir gently with a large wooden spoon to incorporate all ingredients.

Lemon Pasta with Chicken, Cherry Tomatoes and Basil

Ingredients:
- 2 Chicken breasts. diced
- 2 pints Cherry tomatoes
- 4 T Mediterranean olive oil + 2 T if needed
- 2 t Minced garlic
- 24 Fresh basil leaves, diced
- 4 oz. Black olives, sliced
- Himalayan sea salt and coarse ground black pepper to taste
- 1 batch of Lemon Paleo pasta

Instructions:
1. In a large skillet, heat 2T olive oil over medium heat
2. Add diced chicken and cook thoroughly
3. Remove chicken from skillet and set aside
4. Add an additional 2T olive oil and garlic, cook for two minutes
5. Add tomatoes and cook for approximately five minutes, just until they start to soften and burst open, stirring all the while with a wooden spoon to prevent scorching
6. Add diced basil and sliced olives and continue stirring as sauce forms and naturally thickens, adding back in diced chicken
7. Add pasta and if additional olive oil if needed, tossing all ingredients together, sprinkle with salt and pepper to taste
8. Serve and enjoy!

Butternut Squash Pasta with Squash and Ground Turkey

Ingredients:

- 1 lb. Ground turkey
- 1 lb. Butternut squash, diced and steamed
- 2 T + 3 T Mediterranean olive oil
- 2 T Ghee or unsalted butter from grass-fed cows
- ½ Yellow onion, diced
- 2 t Minced garlic
- 1 T Lemon juice
- ½ C Paleo ricotta
- 1 batch of Butternut Squash Paleo pasta

Instructions:

1. Brown ground turkey in 2 T of Mediterranean olive oil in a large skillet over medium heat and remove from pan once browned
2. Add additional 3 T olive oil and ghee or butter to pan with diced onions and garlic and brown over medium heat
3. Add steamed squash and toss lightly
4. Add lemon juice and ricotta, stirring lightly with a wooden spoon
5. Add browned turkey into the vegetable and sauce mixture, stirring with a wooden spoon to incorporate all ingredients
6. Add butternut squash pasta and toss lightly to evenly distribute, heating all ingredients over medium heat and serve!

Chardonnay Pasta with Lobster Fra Diavolo

Ingredients:

- 1/2 t Himalayan sea salt
- 3 medium Lobster tails, broiled, shelled, and chopped
- Pinch Baking soda
- 6 T Mediterranean olive oil
- 3 t Minced garlic
- 1½ t Dried oregano
- 1½ t Red chili flakes
- 1 large can Fire roasted crushed tomatoes
- ½ C Clam juice
- 1 batch of Chardonnay pasta, sliced into spaghetti pasta

Instructions:

1. In a large skillet, heat 4 tablespoons olive oil over medium-high heat, add diced lobster to glaze in olive oil
2. Transfer shrimp to a plate and set aside.
3. Return the skillet to medium-low heat and add garlic, oregano, and chili flakes and cook, stirring, until garlic is just beginning to turn golden, about 2 minutes.
4. Add tomatoes and clam juice and bring to a simmer
5. Add chardonnay spaghetti noodles, and lobster to the sauce, cooking until the sauce reduces and clings to pasta.

Chicken Noodle Soup

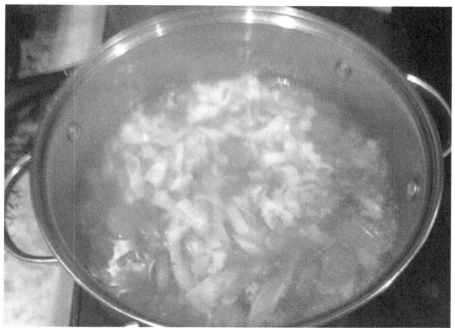

Ingredients:

- 64 oz. Organic chicken bone broth
- 1.5 lbs. Chicken thighs (skinned)
- 10 oz. Carrots, sliced
- 1 t Onion powder
- ½ t Garlic powder
- ½ C Celery, finely sliced
- ½ batch Basic Paleo pasta

Instructions:

1. In a large stock pot, combine broth, chicken, carrots, celery, and spices.
2. Bring to a boil over medium heat, then reduce to simmer for 45 minutes to 1 hour.

3. When chicken is completely cooked and falling off the bones, remove chicken bones and cartilage from soup with a slotted spoon
4. Add pasta and stir gently.

NOTE: You may be tempted to use a full batch of Paleo pasta. However, as the Paleo pasta in a soup base sits, it will absorb the liquid and swell. Therefore, by day two, half a batch of pasta will seem like a full batch is in the soup.

Beef Vegetable Noodle Soup

Ingredients:

- 64 oz. Organic beef bone broth
- 1.5 lbs. Grass-fed tri-tip roast
- 10 oz. Mixed vegetables, diced
- 1 t Onion powder
- ½ t Garlic powder
- ½ batch Tomato pasta

Instructions:

1. In a large stock pot, combine broth, roast, vegetables and spices
2. Bring to a boil over medium heat, then reduce to simmer for 45 minutes to 1 hour.
3. When roast is completely cooked and falling apart, gently break the meat into bite size pieces.
4. Add pasta and stir gently.

NOTE: You may be tempted to use a full batch of Paleo pasta. However, as the Paleo pasta in a soup base sits, it will absorb the liquid and swell. Therefore, by day two, half a batch of pasta will seem like a full batch is in the soup.

Chicken Alfredo

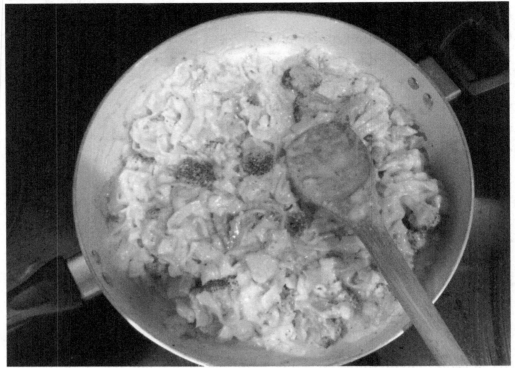

Ingredients:

- 2 T Mediterranean olive oil
- 1.5 lbs. Chicken, cooked and diced
- 10 oz. Broccoli florets, steamed
- 1 batch of Basic Paleo pasta
- 1 batch of Alfredo sauce (recipe in chapter: Sauces and more)

Instructions:

1. Heat olive oil in a large skillet over medium heat
2. Add chicken and broccoli, tossing lightly as they heat
3. Add Alfredo sauce and stir, allow to cook until you see steam, but not boiling.

4. Add pasta and incorporate with a large wooden spoon, continuing to heat until ready to serve!

Turkey Tetrazzini

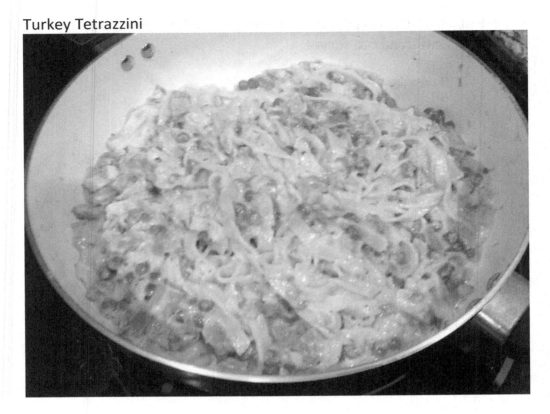

Ingredients:

- 2 T Mediterranean olive oil
- 1.5 lbs. Turkey, cooked and diced
- 10 oz. Petite peas, steamed
- 1 batch of Basic Paleo pasta
- 1 batch of Alfredo sauce (recipe in chapter: Sauces and more)

Instructions:

1. Heat olive oil in a large skillet over medium heat
2. Add turkey and peas, tossing lightly as they heat
3. Add Alfredo sauce and stir, allow to cook until you see steam, but not boiling.

4. Add pasta and incorporate with a large wooden spoon, continuing to heat until ready to serve!

Cold Chicken Pasta Salad

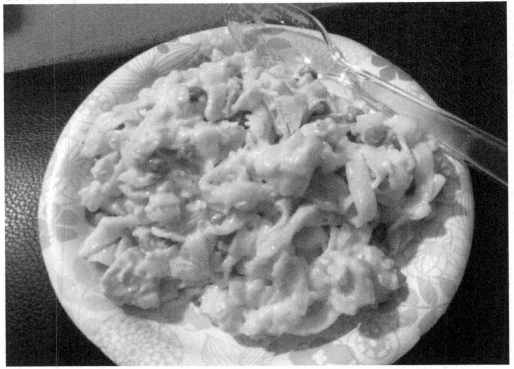

Ingredients:

- 1.5 lb. Chicken breast, cooked, cooled, and diced
- 10 oz. Petite peas, steamed and cooled
- 7 or 8 mini Sweet peppers, mixed
- 1 t Minced garlic (or to taste)
- 1 batch Basic or lemon paleo pasta
- ½ C Paleo avocado mayonnaise

Instructions:

1. Combine chicken, peas, sweet peppers, and garlic in a large bowl, stirring to mix thoroughly
2. Add mayonnaise and mix with a large wooden spoon to combine
3. Add pasta and chill.

Spinach and Avocado with Chicken

Ingredients:
- 1 batch Spinach pasta
- 1 batch Pesto sauce
- 2 Avocados, ripe
- 3 Chicken breasts, diced
- 2 T Mediterranean olive oil
- Lemon zest (optional)

Instructions:
1. In a large skillet heat the olive oil over medium heat. Add the diced chicken and cook thoroughly until insides of diced pieces are no longer pink
2. In a small bowl, combine pesto sauce and avocado, blending together;
3. Add the pesto sauce to the chicken, stir well, and continue heating over medium heat setting.
4. Add the spinach pasta and gently mix with a wooden spoon to distribute pesto sauce throughout
5. Add lemon zest (optional) and toss lightly
6. Once heated, enjoy!

Fall/Winter Cold Pasta Salad

Ingredients:

- 1.5 lbs. chicken breast, cooked, cooled and diced
- 2 Granny smith apples, finely diced
- 1/3 C Paleo dried cranberries
- ½ C Pecans, chopped
- ¼ - ½ t Himalayan sea salt
- ¼ - ½ Ground black pepper (to taste)
- 1 T Extra virgin olive oil
- 2 T Paleo Greek yogurt from grass-fed cows
- ½ C Paleo avocado mayonnaise
- 1 batch Basic or lemon paleo pasta

Instructions:

1. In a large bowl, combine chicken, fruit, nuts, salt, and pepper, stirring to mix thoroughly and set aside
2. In a small bowl, whisk together olive oil, yogurt and mayonnaise
3. Pour mayonnaise mixture over chicken mixture and stir to completely integrate the dressing
4. Add pasta, gently stirring with a large wooden spoon and chill.

Mac and Cheese

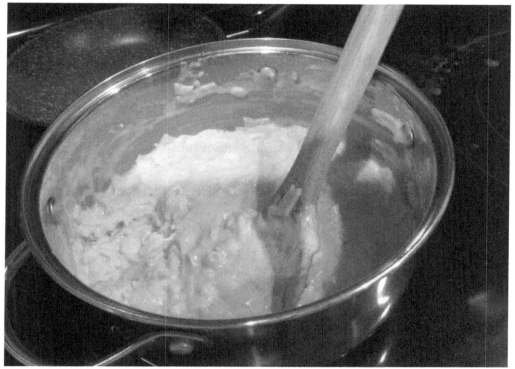

Ingredients:

- ½ wheel (batch) Paleo cheddar cheese (recipe in Sauces... chapter)
- 2 T Coconut cream or almond/coconut milk
- 2 T Ghee or butter from grass-fed cows
- 1 batch Basic Paleo Pasta
- Himalayan sea salt and coarse ground black pepper to taste

Instructions:

1. If you make your pasta with an automated machine, this would be a good recipe with which to use the macaroni disk, but this is optional
2. Once Basic Paleo Pasta has drained, place back in the same pot and return to the stove top over medium heat

3. Add coconut cream or milk and ghee or butter and gently stir with a large wooden spoon, being careful not to damage pasta or macaroni, and let gently come to temperature and reheat
4. In a small bowl, begin melting your Paleo cheddar cheese by placing small strips in the microwave for 15 seconds. You may have to do this several times for half of your cheddar wheel
5. As cheddar cheese melts, pour it directly into the pot with the pasta and gently toss until all cheese has been melted and sauce is thoroughly incorporated
6. Add additional salt, pepper, or even garlic to taste and serve hot.

Bacon Mac and Cheese

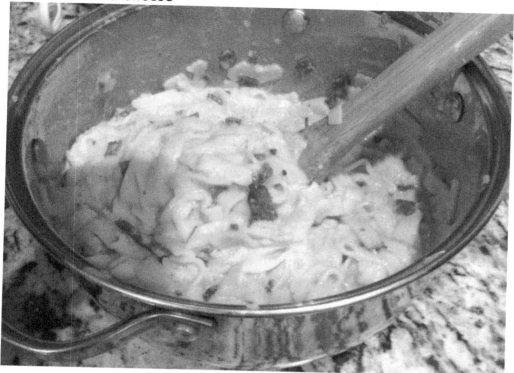

Ingredients:

- 6 strips Paleo Bacon
- ½ wheel (batch) Paleo cheddar cheese (recipe in Sauces... chapter)
- 2 T Coconut cream or almond/coconut milk
- 2 T Ghee or butter from grass-fed cows
- 1 batch Basic Paleo Pasta
- Himalayan sea salt and coarse ground black pepper to taste

Instructions:

1. If you make your pasta with an automated machine, this would be a good recipe with which to use the macaroni disk, but this is optional

2. Start cooking your bacon until crisp, in such a way that allows you to collect some of the bacon grease
3. Once bacon is cooked, allow it to cool, chop into small pieces and set aside
4. Once Basic Paleo Pasta has drained, place back in the same pot and return to the stove top over medium heat
5. Add coconut cream or milk and ghee or butter and gently stir with a large wooden spoon, being careful not to damage pasta or macaroni, and let gently come to temperature and reheat
6. In a small bowl, begin melting your Paleo cheddar cheese by placing small strips in the microwave for 15 seconds. You may have to do this several times for half of your cheddar wheel
7. As cheddar cheese melts, pour it directly into the pot with the pasta and gently toss until all cheese has been melted and sauce is thoroughly incorporated
8. Add bacon pieces and gently stir to mix;
9. Add additional salt, pepper, or even garlic to taste and serve hot.

Tuscan Chicken

Ingredients:

- 1.5 lbs. Chicken breasts, cut in ½ inch strips
- 3 T Mediterranean olive oil
- ¼ C Chicken bone broth up
- 2 t Minced garlic
- 1 t Basil
- 1 t Oregano
- ¼ t Himalayan sea salt
- 1 can Coconut cream
- 2 t Nutritional yeast flakes
- 1 C Baby spinach leaves
- 1/3 C Sun-dried tomatoes, julienne cut
- 1 batch of Basic, lemon, or chardonnay pasta

Option:

Instead of coconut cream, you can use 15 oz. coconut/almond milk and a tapioca flour/cold water slurry to thicken.

Instructions:

1. Heat oil in a large skillet over medium heat
2. While heating oil, place chicken, olive oil, garlic, basil, and oregano in a medium bowl and stir to thoroughly mix to coat chicken
3. Once oil is heated, add chicken strips and cook completely cooked through
4. Once chicken is cooked, add chicken bone broth and nutritional yeast flakes, bringing to a boil. Cook for about 8 minutes
5. Reduce heat to simmer and add coconut cream or coconut/almond milk
6. Bring to a boil and if using coconut/almond milk, add slurry to thicken

7. Add sun dried tomatoes and stir
8. Add fresh baby spinach leaves and stir frequently to incorporate and wilt spinach
9. Add batch of basic, lemon, or chardonnay paleo pasta and stir with a wooden spoon to gently mix

Chapter Eight: Pasta Side Dishes

Lemon Pasta in Garlic Sauce

Ingredients:

- 1 batch Lemon pasta
- ¼ C + 2 T Mediterranean olive oil, divided
- 4 t Minced garlic

Directions

1. In a large skillet, heat ¼ C olive oil
2. Add garlic and cook for 3 minutes
3. Transfer pasta to skillet along with 1/2 cup of the water that the chardonnay pasta cooked in
4. Increase heat to high, and cook, stirring and tossing rapidly, until a creamy, emulsified sauce forms and coats the noodles
5. Remove from heat, add remaining 2 tablespoons olive oil, toss to combine, and serve right away.

Lemon Pasta with Asparagus and Peas

Ingredients:

- ½ batch of Lemon pasta
- ½ batch of Lemon cashew sauce (recipe in Sauces and more section)
- 12 Asparagus spears, steamed
- 8 oz. Petite peas, steamed

Instructions:

1. Combine sauce and vegetables in a large skillet over medium heat
2. Add pasta, and gently mix with a large wooden spoon tossing lightly
3. Serve when thoroughly heated

Sweet Potato Cinnamon Pasta

Ingredients:

- ¼ C Ghee or butter from grass fed cows, melted
- 2 t Vietnamese cinnamon
- 1 T Palm sugar
- 1/2 batch Sweet potato pasta

Instructions:

1. Combine ghee/butter, cinnamon, and sugar in a large skillet over medium heat and whisk together
2. Add sweet potato pasta and gently mix with a large wooden spoon tossing lightly.
3. Serve when thoroughly heated.

Butter Herb Pasta

Ingredients:
- ½ batch Basic pasta
- ¼ C Melted ghee or butter from grass fed cows
- 2 T Mediterranean olive oil
- 2 t Minced garlic
- 2 t Oregano

Instructions:
1. In a large skillet, combine melted ghee or butter, olive oil, garlic, and oregano over medium heat. Whisk to thoroughly combine all ingredients
2. Add cold or hot basic pasta, and toss lightly
3. Serve

Antipasti Pasta

Ingredients:

- 1 T Oregano
- 1 T Lemon juice
- ¼ C Mediterranean olive oil
- 1/2 batch Basic, tomato, or spinach pasta
- ½ Red onion, finely diced
- ¼ C Black olives, sliced
- 20 thinly sliced piece of Paleo pepperoni or Italian Sausage

Instructions:

1. Combine oregano, lemon juice, and olive oil in a large mixing bowl, and whisk until a thick dressing is formed.
2. Combine cold or hot basic, tomato, or spinach pasta and remaining ingredients in a medium mixing bowl, gently mixing with a large wooden spoon to protect the integrity of the pasta
3. Pour dressing over pasta and vegetable mixture, and toss lightly.
4. Serve

Greek Beet Pasta Side
Ingredients:
- 1 T Oregano
- 1 T Thyme
- 1 T Lemon juice
- ¼ C Mediterranean olive oil
- 1/2 batch Beet pasta
- ½ Red onion, finely diced
- ¼ C Kalamata olives, finely diced
- 1/3 C Feta cheese (if following a Lacto-Paleo diet)

Instructions:
1. Combine oregano, thyme, lemon juice, and olive oil in a small mixing bowl, and whisk until a thick dressing is formed.
2. Combine cold or hot beet pasta and remaining ingredients in a medium mixing bowl, gently mixing with a large wooden spoon to protect the integrity of the pasta
3. Pour dressing over pasta and vegetable mixture, and toss lightly.
4. Serve

Creamed Spinach Pasta

Ingredients:

- ½ batch Spinach pasta
- 2 t Minced garlic
- 1 can Full fat coconut cream
- 1/4 t Nutmeg
- large pinch Himalayan sea salt
- Black pepper to taste
- 2 T Ghee
- 1 T Mediterranean olive oil

Instructions:

1. In a large skillet combine the ghee and olive oil over medium heat. Add the garlic and sauté until fragrant, about 30 seconds.
2. Add the coconut cream and add the nutmeg, salt and pepper. Bring the mixture to a low simmer.
3. Add the spinach pasta and gently mix with a wooden spoon to distribute cream sauce throughout
4. Continue to simmer until sauce has thickened and the liquid has reduced by half. Enjoy!

Chardonnay Pasta with Lemon and Asparagus

Ingredients:

- ½ batch Chardonnay pasta
- ½ batch Lemon cashew sauce
- 12 Asparagus spears, steamed and cut into 1" pieces
- 1 T Extra virgin olive oil

Instructions:

1. In a large skillet heat the olive oil over medium heat. Add the sliced asparagus and sauté for about 2 minutes
2. Add the lemon cashew cream and bring the mixture to a low simmer.
3. Add the chardonnay pasta and gently mix with a wooden spoon to distribute cream sauce throughout
4. Once heated, enjoy!

Chapter Nine: Pasta Desserts

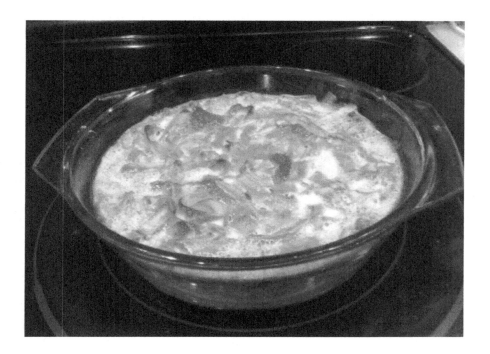

Strawberries and Cream
Ingredients:

- 6 Eggs
- ½ C Almond or almond coconut milk
- 1/3 C Fruit sweet
- 1 batch Strawberry pasta
- 1 C sliced Ripe strawberries in season (alt: 1/3 C Paleo strawberry preserves)

Instructions:

1. Preheat oven to 350 degrees
2. Lightly grease a lasagna pan with coconut oil, especially up the sides
3. In a very large bowl, combine eggs, coconut/almond milk, and fruit sweet
4. Add strawberry pasta and gently stir with a wooden spoon
5. Add preserves of fresh strawberries and stir again being gentle with the pasta
6. Once all is thoroughly blended, poor into your prepared lasagna pan
7. Bake for 45 minutes or until center is just set and edges are slightly browned.

Strawberries and Lemon Custard
Ingredients:
- 6 Eggs
- ½ C Almond or almond coconut milk
- 1/3 C Fruit sweet
- ¼ C Fresh lemon juice
- 1 batch Strawberry pasta
- 1 C sliced Ripe strawberries in season (alt: 1/3 C Paleo strawberry preserves)

Instructions:
1. Preheat oven to 350 degrees
2. Lightly grease a lasagna pan with coconut oil, especially up the sides
3. In a very large bowl, combine eggs, coconut/almond milk, lemon juice, and fruit sweet
4. Add strawberry pasta and gently stir with a wooden spoon
5. Add preserves of fresh strawberries and stir again being gentle with the pasta
6. Once all is thoroughly blended, poor into your prepared lasagna pan
7. Bake for 45 minutes or until center is just set and edges are slightly browned.

Tropical Custard

Ingredients:

- 6 Eggs
- ½ C Almond or almond coconut milk
- 1/3 C Fruit sweet
- 1 batch Basic pasta
- ¾ C Shredded unsweetened coconut flakes
- ¾ C Mandarin orange slices
- ¾ C Crushed pineapple

Instructions:

1. Preheat oven to 350 degrees
2. Lightly grease a lasagna pan with coconut oil, especially up the sides
3. In a very large bowl, combine eggs, coconut/almond milk, and fruit sweet
4. Add basic Paleo pasta and gently stir with a wooden spoon
5. Add shredded coconut, mandarin oranges, and pineapple stirring gently with a wooden spoon
6. Once all is thoroughly blended, poor into your prepared lasagna pan
7. Bake for 45 minutes or until center is just set and edges are slightly browned.

Bananas Dolce La Leche
Ingredients:
- 6 Eggs
- ½ C Almond or almond coconut milk
- 1/3 C Fruit sweet
- 1 batch Banana pasta
- 1 Ripe banana

Instructions:
1. Preheat oven to 350 degrees
2. Lightly grease a lasagna pan with coconut oil, especially up the sides
3. In a food processor, puree banana (alt: mash banana in a bowl, assuring no chunks)
4. In a very large bowl, combine eggs, coconut/almond milk, banana, and fruit sweet
5. Add banana pasta and gently stir with a wooden spoon
6. Once all is thoroughly blended, poor into your prepared lasagna pan
7. Bake for 45 minutes or until center is just set and edges are slightly browned.

Coffee and Chocolate Custard

Ingredients:

- 6 Eggs
- ½ C Almond or almond coconut milk
- 1/3 C Fruit sweet
- 1 batch Coffee pasta
- 3 T Dutch cocoa powder
- ½ C Paleo chocolate chips (optional)

Instructions:

1. Preheat oven to 350 degrees
2. Lightly grease a lasagna pan with coconut oil, especially up the sides
3. In a very large bowl, combine eggs, coconut/almond milk, cocoa powder, and fruit sweet
4. Add coffee Paleo pasta and gently stir with a wooden spoon
5. Add Paleo chocolate chips if using
6. Once all is thoroughly blended, poor into your prepared lasagna pan
7. Bake for 45 minutes or until center is just set and edges are slightly browned.

Merlot and Chocolate Sauce

Ingredients:

- 6 Eggs
- ½ C Almond or almond coconut milk
- 1/3 C Fruit sweet
- 1 batch Merlot pasta
- 3 T Dutch cocoa powder
- ½ C Paleo chocolate chips (optional)

Instructions:

1. Preheat oven to 350 degrees
2. Lightly grease a lasagna pan with coconut oil, especially up the sides
3. In a very large bowl, combine eggs, coconut/almond milk, cocoa powder, and fruit sweet
4. Add merlot Paleo pasta and gently stir with a wooden spoon
5. Add Paleo chocolate chips if using
6. Once all is thoroughly blended, poor into your prepared lasagna pan
7. Bake for 45 minutes or until center is just set and edges are slightly browned.

Triple Chocolate Pasta Dessert

Ingredients:

- 6 Eggs
- ½ C Almond or almond coconut milk
- 1/3 C Fruit sweet
- 1 batch Chocolate pasta
- 3 T Dutch cocoa powder
- ½ C Paleo chocolate chips (optional)

Instructions:

1. Preheat oven to 350 degrees
2. Lightly grease a lasagna pan with coconut oil, especially up the sides
3. In a very large bowl, combine eggs, coconut/almond milk, cocoa powder, and fruit sweet
4. Add merlot Paleo pasta and gently stir with a wooden spoon
5. Add Paleo chocolate chips if using
6. Once all is thoroughly blended, poor into your prepared lasagna pan
7. Bake for 45 minutes or until center is just set and edges are slightly browned.

Strawberries and Chocolate Sauce
Ingredients:
- 6 Eggs
- ½ C Almond or almond coconut milk
- 1/3 C Fruit sweet
- 1 batch Strawberry pasta
- 3 T Dutch cocoa powder
- ½ C Paleo chocolate chips (optional)

Instructions:
1. Preheat oven to 350 degrees
2. Lightly grease a lasagna pan with coconut oil, especially up the sides
3. In a very large bowl, combine eggs, coconut/almond milk, cocoa powder, and fruit sweet
4. Add coffee strawberry pasta and gently stir with a wooden spoon
5. Add Paleo chocolate chips if using
6. Once all is thoroughly blended, poor into your prepared lasagna pan
7. Bake for 45 minutes or until center is just set and edges are slightly browned.

Chardonnay and Strawberry Sauce
Ingredients:

- 6 Eggs
- ½ C Almond or almond coconut milk
- 1/3 C Fruit sweet
- 1 batch Chardonnay pasta
- 1/3 C Strawberry preserves
- 1 C sliced Ripe fresh strawberries (optional)

Instructions:

1. Preheat oven to 350 degrees
2. Lightly grease a lasagna pan with coconut oil, especially up the sides
3. In a very large bowl, combine eggs, coconut/almond milk, strawberry preserves, and fruit sweet
4. Add chardonnay Paleo pasta and gently stir with a wooden spoon
5. Add fresh strawberries if using
6. Once all is thoroughly blended, poor into your prepared lasagna pan
7. Bake for 45 minutes or until center is just set and edges are slightly browned.

About the Author

Dr. West-Stellick is a much sought after naturopath with clients literally throughout the world. When not working directly with clients, Dr. West is a well-respected writer, lecturer, seminar leader, and culinary sleuth!

After spending upwards of 30 years in corporate America in a variety of management positions, Dr. West-Stellick's passion for medicine overcame her business success and she received a doctorate of natural healthcare, establishing and maintaining a very successful practice for 17 years, subsequently spending another 10 years as a medical ghostwriter and researcher. Dr. West is the author of over 25 books on a wide variety of topics, for both the secular and Christian market, including: *Ten Essential and Simple Steps to Managing Your Doctor: Empowering you, the Patient; Ten Essential and Simple Steps to Becoming Your Own Case Manager: A Guide for Handling Multiple Medical Issues; Authentic, Inspired, Inerrant, and True; In Sickness and in Health; God, Marriage, and Illness; The God Prescription; Fear of Forgetting Jesus; My Life, My Memories; Preventing Dementia Naturally: Assuring the healthy child, adult, and senior throughout the generations; Paleo Basics: A delicious guide to what Paleo is all about, and how to become a Paleo Pro in no time!, Paleo Pasta: The Art of Making Amazing Paleo, Grain-Free, and Gluten-Free Pasta, and The Paleo Pup!*

Other Lariat Publishing Books by Dr. Danielle West-Stellick

Ten Essential and Simple Steps to Managing Your Doctor: Empowering you, the Patient

Ten Essential and Simple Steps to Managing your Doctor: Empowering You, the Patient provides a wealth of information in easy to follow segments that will transition you from being the passive patient to the empowered patient, from waiting and being at the mercy of the medical system to the patient who takes responsibility for their healthcare and their life as they seek to form a partnership with their physician. The Ten Essential and Simple Steps to Managing Your Doctor: Empowering You, the Patient is written in an easy to follow workbook format, including pages you can scan or photocopy and use as is or adapt for your own use. For other situations discussed, such as reaching your physician when you have questions or even emergency situations and need to speak with him, sample scenarios are written out in script fashion, providing the framework for your own adaptation to your specific situations as needed. ISBN: 978-1887219211

Ten Essential and Simple Steps to Becoming Your Own Case Manager: A Guide for Handling Multiple Medical Issues

Keeping track of one health issue is sometimes enough to make a person crazy! Juggling multiple health challenges can be impossible! The ten very simple steps in this book help you become your own case manager, help you organize and keep track each illness and the doctors involved. The steps in this book also helps you maintain a position of authority and strength while assuring all doctors involved in each piece of the puzzle that is uniquely you, are communicating effectively with a complete and comprehensive flow of information among and between all parties providing any level of care for you. This is in workbook format, inclusive of forms and pages you may wish to scan or photocopy and use. ISBN: 978-1887219228

Authentic, Inspired, Inerrant, and True

From the beginning, Satan has attempted to make us question God's Word to us. Part of Satan's plan is to cause us to doubt that the Bible is God's authentic, inspired, inerrant and true message to us all. It's easier to look at the Bible as a storybook or piece of literature rather than know God's Word is the truth. Thus, many people think of the Bible as a storybook of a book of historical literature - therefore, whether it is true or not is immaterial. Many people say they believe in parts of the Bible, but not others. We know that the Bible is authentic, inspired, inerrant and true Word of God: if part is true, all is true. If all of God's word is true, we must face the truth about our own moral character. Thus, through independent research and with the goal of Scripture proving Scripture rather than relying on what man says about God's Word, this book gradually came together exploring such topics as: what God says, statistical proof, historical and archeological evidence, and prophecy. And finally, we look at how the various versions of the Bible came about and a candid discussion is provided on how accurate or inaccurate they today's Bibles are. Let Dr. West-Stellick lead you on an exciting journal that lays the foundation, and then covers 3,500 years of writing, translations, discoveries and more. *Authentic, Inspired, Inerrant and True* will bring you to the fact-based conclusion: The Bible IS God's Word to us. ISBN: 978-1887219105

In Sickness and in Health

In Sickness and in Health represents raw emotion. Inside you will find friends who have experienced what happens when chronic illness becomes the uninvited third member in your marital relationship. Inside, patients share their stories of pain and regret; partners and spouses share their frustrations, and fears. Both share the experiences of unplanned changes to their relationship. All share stories that are all too common when people gloss over the "In Sickness and in Health" part of their wedding vows, and reality sets in when someone is diagnosed with a life-altering chronic illness. This book provides a key message to all patients and partners: you are not alone. Others have walked (or been wheeled) in your shoes. *In Sickness and in Health* provides the unique ability to learn what your partner is likely to be thinking and why he or she is behaving in a specific way that you may not know about. This book does not promise to transform your relationship, but it does promise to leave you with the knowledge that you are not alone in your journey. ISBN: 978-1887219204

God, Marriage, and Illness

It is a sobering truth. The divorce rate for physically healthy couples is between 40-50 %, the divorce rate for those plagued by chronic illness is in excess of 75 percent. When illness strikes, suddenly most people wonder what happened to that wonderful, caring, sensitive person they fell in love with. They wonder why they feel alone, and why they hurt even though they are still married or in a significant relationship. They wonder why their Godly marriage is falling apart. Part of the problem is focus. When there is a lack of reliance on God once illness presents in a marriage, the Illness, Marriage, and God paradigm needs to be transformed into one that places God first, followed by your marriage, and then, and only then, the focus on illness should enter into the triad. With the rate of chronic illnesses increasing at an alarming rate, readers must take action and INVEST to protect or repair their marriage in only the way that dependence and a focus on God can provide! What *God, Marriage, and Illness* offers is an interactive workbook designed to enable the reader a way to regain the proper perspective and focus on God first in their life. ISBN: 978-188721920242

The God Prescription
Despite professional medical evidence that stresses prayer and attention to the spiritual life of a chronically ill patient dramatically serves to improve their quality of life, upwards of 72% of all healthcare professionals never broach the subject with their patients, opting to focus instead on the medical model of patient care. Sadly, the traditional medical model draws the patient's attention away from the spiritual Godly realm and focuses it on the patient themselves. The real focus need to remain on Him, not the self. *The God Prescription* puts the focus back on God. *The God Prescription* can help you to: 1. Enhance your quality of life; 2. Reduce chronic pain and inflammation; 3. Transform limitations into opportunities that glorify God; and 4. Draw you closer to God. Writing from personal experience as a doctor and as a patient, Dr. West brings you: *The God Prescription.* ISBN: 978-1887219020

Fear of Forgetting Jesus
Building on the Christian edition of *Fear of Forgetting*, which delves into the heart and soul of a person diagnosed with Alzheimer's disease or one of the dementias as virtually every area of their life is examined. Following a detailed presentation of the physiology involved in the disease progression, with the help of scripture, areas of the individual's life are examined along with probing questions requiring the patient to document their feelings and experiences, along with their questions regarding risks, how they feel about memory loss and issues related to making new memories, including a major section delving into

who the patient thinks Jesus is, their relationship with Jesus, familial history and experiences, favorite prayers, favorite scriptures, and more. A detailed exploration of generational curses and sin are also incorporated, as is a strong focus on prayer and the development of a prayer life that can transcend their journey. Like *Fear of Forgetting*, *Fear of Forgetting Jesus* guides the reader past their diagnosis and provides important information in an easy to understand way that educates the patient about what is really happening to their brain, what the journey will be like, and what they can do about their diagnosis to embrace their journey. *Fear of Forgetting Jesus* is also purposely designed to enable easy reading for the older individual already in the early stages of the disease; in workbook format, it guides the patient through an introspective process of examining and documenting their fears, thoughts, and emotions about the diagnosis, the journey they will take, and *how they believe it will be best to reach them* as the disease progresses based on their unique life events, likes, and dislike, and should become a living journal for family and friends to use as a non-threatening springboard for discussion and care. And like *Fear of Forgetting*, *Fear of Forgetting Jesus* also includes the free bonus: *My Life, My Memories*, a special memory prompting diary all about who you are! ISBN: 978-1887219273

My Life, My Memories

My Life, My Memories is a journal for completion by the dementia patient This journal will prompt you to write out answers to questions about your life, and your memories. The goal is to achieve a comprehensive book of your life, who you are, and what you are most likely to remember most as Alzheimer's disease or one of the other dementias progress. This journal will tie the patient's current life and past (stored memories) together. It will also help others to work with the patient in the later stages of the disease when, based on the patient's responses to the prompts in this book, for example, when you state likes and dislikes not only from the present but from the past. Topics covered include general information (such as your name), work history, education, romance, childhood and teen years, religion, food, and a section called "last but not least" where the patient can enter anything else that may have been overlooked but is considered by the patient to be important! ISBN: 978-1887219327

Paleo Basics: A delicious guide to what Paleo is all about, and how to become a Paleo Pro in no time!

Paleo Basics is designed to provide a wealth of information on the why's and how-to's of starting on the Paleo Diet, filling in many of the gaps left in other books. For example, in Part One, *Paleo Basics* starts out explaining what the Paleo Diet is, and why a person should follow it, then goes on to discuss the finer points one needs to know in order to really make the Paleo Diet a lifestyle change. For example, setting up the Paleo kitchen, what is a Paleo grocery list like and how to construct one, how to grocery shop, and so forth. Then we talk about how to maintain a social life and remain on the Paleo Diet. Part Two picks up with super easy, delicious, and versatile recipes ranging from appetizers and breakfast dishes to sauces, snacks, and baked goods. This book is a must have to answer all the most common questions about going Paleo, and more than that, guides you through easy Paleo recipes that will ensure you can become a Paleo Pro in no time at all!

ISBN: 978-1887219471

The Paleo Pup

More and more and more veterinarians and veterinary bloggers are advocating raw and grain-free diets for their dog. As a result, healthful dog food and dog treat manufacturers are supplying raw and grain-free products. With this in mind, Part One of T*he Paleo Pup* examines the health issues surrounding raw and grain-free feeding, and Part Two provides a wide raw and grain-free recipes to delight your pet! ISBN: 978-1887219495

Paleo Pasta!

Consultations provided worldwide via Skype. Please leave a message on my Facebook page link below.

Be sure to LIKE us on Facebook:

https://www.facebook.com/Dr-Danielle-West-ND-Naturopathic-Healthcare-201497746608979/

All publications are available on Amazon throughout the world!

Made in the USA
Middletown, DE
13 December 2019